THE DELL
NATURAL MEDICINE LIBRARY

NATURAL MEDICINE FOR
WEIGHT LOSS

Deborah Mitchell

Foreword by P. Scott Ricke, M.D.

A Lynn Sonberg Book

A Dell Book

Published by
Dell Publishing
a division of
Bantam Doubleday Dell Publishing Group, Inc.
1540 Broadway
New York, New York 10036

IMPORTANT NOTE: Neither this nor any other book should be used as a substitute for professional medical care or treatment. It is advisable to seek the guidance of a physician or other qualified health practitioner before implementing any of the approaches to health suggested in this book. This book was written to provide selected information to the public concerning conventional and alternative medical treatments for weight loss. Research in this field is ongoing and subject to interpretation. Although we have made all reasonable efforts to include the most up-to-date and accurate information in this book, there is no guarantee that what we know about this complex subject won't change with time. The reader should bear in mind that this book is not intended to take the place of medical advice from a trained medical professional. Readers are advised to consult a physician or other qualified health professional regarding treatment of all of their health problems. Neither the publisher, the producer nor the authors take any responsibility for any possible consequences from any treatment, action or application of medicine or preparation by any person reading or following the information in this book. The patients depicted in this book are composites and do not represent any one individual.

ISBN: 0-440-22522-1

Published by arrangement with
Lynn Sonberg Book Associates
10 West 86th Street
New York, NY 10024

Printed in the United States of America

Published simultaneously in Canada

July 1998

10 9 8 7 6 5 4 3 2 1

OPM

CONTENTS

FOREWORD

One thing I am most committed to in medicine is forever altering the perception that overweight people are that way on purpose; that they are overweight because they are "fat and lazy," or they "lack discipline." One of the myths of our culture is that obesity is a disease of willpower rather than a complex metabolic or endocrine disorder.

There is no other medical condition that is more shrouded in misconceptions, inaccurate information, stereotypical thinking, and just plain mean-spirited accusations than obesity. How many times have you overheard someone look at an overweight person and say that they have done it to themselves, that they don't care how they look, or why don't they just "exercise more and just say 'no' to food?" How many of those same thoughts have you had yourself or about yourself?

Such moral overlays might be useful if obesity were a theological dilemma. How many overweight people have been made to feel guilty or shameful about their weight? Did that ever produce the desired result? If being overweight is a simple problem of willpower, then why are overweight people unable to will themselves thin?

The reason is not that they are unwilling; it is because they are unable. Since there is no medical benefit to being overweight, to imply that over 100 million obese people in this country actually will themselves to be overweight, or that they are happy about it, is implausible and defies logic. They may be resigned to it, perhaps even accept it, but never happy about it. Ask any adult if they like being overweight; ask any child.

Like other metabolic and endocrine disorders, obesity is a disease that may be inherited, chronic, active, progressive, and lethal. More than 300,000 people die every year from the direct effects of being overweight. Fatal strokes, heart attacks, and cancer interfere with a long and fruitful life.

To date, researchers have identified at least seven different genes and ten different hormones that are associated with being overweight. Maybe we can start to look at overweight as a symptom of an untreated medical condition rather than a character flaw.

We view diabetes and other endocrine disorders as medical conditions that are worthy to be treated medically, yet not obesity. No one has an objection to a diabetic person taking insulin. It's helpful to understand that an overweight person suffers from food cravings for salt- or sugar-based foods, and they do not experience normal fullness. This leads to overeating and *involuntary weight gain*. These food cravings are uncontrollable. Overweight people can no more control their appetite than diabetics can control their blood sugar by willpower alone. Diabetics do not need to be lectured or given a lesson in morality, they need insulin. Give them that and they get better.

As with diabetes, the medical literature clearly indicates that when overweight people are treated, they get better. This book addresses the vast amount of research that has been conducted in the field of natural medicine that provides overweight people with tools, and a better understanding of what has been going on for most, if not all, their lives.

Natural Medicine for Weight Loss succeeds in giving people information and options that allow them to make a choice. Either they start managing the disease, albeit imperfectly, or they allow the disease to continue to manage them.

People can effectively use tools if they understand how to use them. This book gives people access to taking back some control of their lives, at least when it comes to addressing obesity.

The material contained in this comprehensive book is important because people need all the information available in order to make informed choices regarding their approach to weight loss. This is an excellent reference for a wide range of natural treatment modalities. It is well researched and well thought out, and it gives the reader useful information grounded in the literature, distinct from someone's personal opinion about the subject.

Finally, the disease of obesity can start to be seen through a different filter: a medical filter through which overweight people can start to be appropriately treated rather than inappropriately judged.

P. Scott Ricke, M.D.
Director
The Institute for Medical Weight Loss
Tucson, Arizona

INTRODUCTION

You know diets don't work. You know because you've probably tried a few, perhaps dozens. They don't work because they don't offer you workable, positive, long-term tools and goals to help you lose weight and keep it off, safely and healthily. They leave you hungry and unsatisfied. Most of them don't help you understand the reason why you are overweight or why you overeat, or help you understand how your mind and body are intimately connected in your quest for a thinner, healthier you. Sure, you can lose 5 or 10 pounds in a week or two by eating just grapefruit or by taking diet pills. But you cannot live on grapefruit or diet pills for the rest of your life . . . nor would you want to! And with the controversies and recalls concerning diet drugs—including the recall of phen-fen and Redux because of the apparent link with valvular heart problems and primary pulmonary hypertension—using natural weight loss methods becomes ever more appealing.

Even the word *diet* sounds depressing and negative. *Diet* brings to mind deprivation, starving, fasting, celery and carrots, hunger pangs, uncontrollable cravings . . . unpleasant thoughts and feelings, to be sure. As if these things weren't enough, we live in a society that places extraordinary pressure, especially on women, to be thin. The media message is thin = beauty, success, acceptance, which is not only unfair but untrue.

Thus, if you want an affirming, healthy, enjoyable, and

satisfying way not only to shed pounds but to acquire a positive attitude about yourself and how you look and feel, this is the book for you. This book is about making healthy, nondrug, natural choices concerning weight loss. Not only does it help you develop a healthy relationship with food, physical activity, and your body; it also gives you the information you need to incorporate weight loss "helpers and boosters" into your life. There are dozens of herbs, nutrients, supplements, and natural medicine techniques that can help make losing weight easier and safe. This book helps you choose among some of the more effective holistic approaches that facilitate weight loss. Combined with the latest information and tips on nutrition and stress-reducing, life-affirming activities also contained in these pages, you can soon be on the path of a positive weight loss experience. You'll learn how your body and mind work together to create the person you are now and the person you want to be: lighter physically, lighter in spirit, and empowered with energy. Once you do, you'll realize that you can lose weight and be healthy, confident, poised, and successful—without the need to look like a fashion model.

Weight control is a lifetime commitment. The eating plan you adopt and other steps you take to help you stay on course should be things you can follow for a lifetime. They should make you feel fulfilled in body, mind, and spirit. A 500-calorie liquid diet may help you lose a few pounds quickly, but it is not something you can continue. And in addition to the havoc most diets cause in the body, statistics show that most people regain the weight they lose, and often even more pounds than they shed.

If this book were the standard "Eat Less, Exercise More" tome about weight loss, you could toss it on the pile with the hundreds of other volumes that help people count calories and give pep talks on how to exercise more. If it claimed to have the "magic formula" or the "secret pill" for losing weight fast and without effort, you could throw it on the mountain of books and literature that make such fantastic claims. But *Natural Medicine for Weight Loss* fits into neither of those categories. It recognizes that losing weight is not about willpower—it's about changing thought processes and the way people think about themselves. It's about taking advantage of the natural herbs, nutrients, and techniques that can help them make losing weight—and maintaining the loss—easier.

You probably recognize the formula for weight loss: Eat Fewer Calories + Exercise = Weight Loss. This equation does not take into consideration the many wonderful, natural aids available to people who want to lose weight. That's why *our* equation reads: Good Dietary Habits + Enjoyable Exercise + Positive Mind-Body Reinforcement + Nature's Helpers = Permanent Weight Loss. In this book we not only explain how the natural approaches work; we also discuss, in depth, the weight loss programs of three individuals who integrated holistic concepts into their lives. They used the new equation and it worked for them. It can work for you, too.

For a few people, medication use or physical disabilities may be factors in their being overweight. Increasing evidence also suggests that genetics plays a role in people's ability to lose or gain weight. Regardless of the factors involved in your challenge to lose weight, you have an incredible tool at your disposal—your mind-body—and as you nurture it you will develop a lighter, healthier, and more wholesome way of eating and being.

PART ONE

WHY AMERICA IS GAINING WEIGHT

CHAPTER ONE

Weight Loss and Gain: What's It All About

You want to lose weight. You're tired of playing games, feeling hungry, wasting your time and money, and regaining any weight you've lost. You don't want drugs or any more broken promises. You've heard and read the weight loss ads that sound too good to be true . . . and they are. Now you want straight talk about weight loss. You want to feel good about the way you look. You want to be in control of your weight. Before you can take back control—or perhaps have control for the first time in your life—you need to know where you stand.

Overweight in America: Where We Stand

Every year, millions of Americans make a tremendous investment. According to the National Academy of Sciences Institute of Medicine, Americans spend more than $33 billion annually on weight loss programs and diet aids, such as protein drinks or foods. For that investment, they reap dubious dividends: the vast majority of people will eventually gain back all the weight they lost, plus a few extra pounds.

That's a good return if you're investing in the stock market; not so good if you are a dieter. The National Institutes of Health (NIH) report that of people who enroll in organized weight-loss programs, 95 percent will regain two-thirds of the pounds they lose within one to three years. So while the media saturates the public with the idea that they must be thin, the only things losing weight are consumers' wallets.

The paradox is that for all their efforts to lose weight, Americans are getting fatter. Between 1980 and 1994, the proportion of overweight adults increased 9 percent; among children and adolescents, the increase was 6 percent. The results of the third National Health and Nutrition Examination Survey (NHANES), conducted 1988–1994, show that the percentage of people who are overweight is approximately 14 percent among children aged 6 to 11; 12 percent of adolescents aged 12 to 17; and 35 percent of adults 20 years and older. Translation: One in three, or 58 million American adults aged 20 through 74 are overweight. A closer look reveals that minority populations edge out whites: approximately 50 percent of black or Hispanic women are overweight.

Millions of Americans say they are on a diet. The percentage of adult American women trying to lose weight at any given time is 33 to 40 percent; among men, 20 to 24 percent. Information about diets and weight loss programs abounds, yet most of it is wrapped up in so much hype and false promises that Americans are still misinformed and misled about dieting and weight loss. One result is that many individuals set unrealistic goals and become discouraged when their hoped-for weight loss does not occur. Another is that some people do not acknowledge their obesity or choose to deny that their overweight is a problem.

Are You Overweight?

Not all physicians and dietary experts agree on the exact definitions of *overweight* and *obesity,* but a general consensus has been reached. The word *overweight* means an excess amount of body weight, which includes bone, fat, water, and muscle. *Obesity* is the excess accumulation of body fat. Doctors and scientists generally agree that individuals are clinically obese if they are 20 percent or more above their desirable weight.

Measuring Body Mass and Body Fat

Scientists devised the Body Mass Index (BMI) as a tool to help classify individuals as overweight or obese. Physicians and obesity researchers prefer the BMI to other methods (which are described below). Body mass index is determined by dividing a person's weight in kilograms by height in meters squared. Men with a BMI greater than 27.8 and women with a BMI greater than 27.3 are considered obese. Or to put it another way, a man who is six feet tall and weighs 210 pounds and a woman who is five feet two inches and weighs 150 pounds are obese, according to this formula. Most Americans who are overweight have a BMI of 27 to 30, which is "mildly obese." These people are about 20 to 40 pounds heavier than their ideal weight. An estimated 41 percent of the population have a BMI of 25.1 or higher, and 8 percent have a BMI of 35 and greater, which is classified as severely obese.

You can determine your own BMI by using the following chart. It has already converted the centimeters and kilograms into inches and pounds for you. Find the intersection of your height and weight and you will have your BMI.

Physicians often depend on weight-for-height tables as a guideline to classify someone as obese. Unfortunately, there are many different versions of these tables. Some factor in

Body Mass Index Chart

Height Weight lb	4'10"	4'11"	5'	5'1"	5'2"	5'3"	5'4"	5'5"	5'6"	5'7"	5'8"
100	20.9	20.2	19.6	18.9	18.3	17.8	17.2	16.7	16.2	15.7	15.2
110	23.0	22.3	21.5	20.8	20.2	19.5	18.9	18.3	17.8	17.3	16.8
120	25.1	24.3	23.5	22.7	22.0	21.3	20.6	20.0	19.4	18.8	18.3
130	27.2	26.3	25.4	24.6	23.8	23.1	22.4	21.7	21.0	20.4	19.8
140	29.3	28.3	27.4	26.5	25.7	24.9	24.1	23.3	22.6	22.0	21.3
150	31.4	30.4	29.4	28.4	27.5	26.6	25.8	25.0	24.3	23.5	22.9
160	33.5	32.4	31.3	30.3	29.3	28.4	27.5	26.7	25.9	25.1	24.4
170	35.6	34.4	33.3	32.2	31.2	30.2	29.2	28.3	27.5	26.7	25.9
180	37.7	36.4	35.2	34.1	33.0	32.0	31.0	30.0	29.1	28.3	27.4
190	39.8	38.5	37.2	36.0	34.8	33.7	32.7	31.7	30.7	29.8	28.9
200	41.9	40.5	39.1	37.9	36.7	35.5	34.4	33.4	32.3	31.4	30.5
205	42.9	41.5	40.1	38.8	37.6	36.4	35.3	34.2	33.2	32.2	31.2
210	44.0	42.5	41.1	39.8	38.5	37.3	36.1	35.0	34.0	33.0	32.0
215	45.0	43.5	42.1	40.7	39.4	38.2	37.0	35.9	34.8	33.7	32.8
220	46.1	44.5	43.1	41.7	40.3	39.1	37.8	36.7	35.6	34.5	33.5
225	47.1	45.5	44.0	42.6	41.2	39.9	38.7	37.5	36.4	35.3	34.3
230	48.2	46.6	45.0	43.5	42.2	40.8	39.6	38.4	37.2	36.1	35.0
235	49.2	47.6	46.0	44.5	43.1	41.7	40.4	39.2	38.0	36.9	35.8
240	50.3	48.6	47.0	45.4	44.0	42.6	41.3	40.0	38.8	37.7	36.6
245	51.3	49.6	47.9	46.4	44.9	43.5	42.1	40.9	39.6	38.5	37.3
250	52.4	50.6	48.9	47.3	45.8	44.4	43.0	41.7	40.4	39.2	38.1
255	53.4	51.6	49.9	48.3	46.7	45.3	43.9	42.5	41.2	40.0	38.9
260	54.5	52.6	50.9	49.2	47.7	46.2	44.7	43.4	42.1	40.8	38.6
265	55.5	53.6	51.9	50.2	48.6	47.0	45.6	44.2	42.9	41.6	40.4
270	56.5	54.6	52.8	51.1	49.5	47.9	46.4	45.0	43.7	42.4	41.1
275	57.6	55.7	53.8	52.1	50.4	48.8	47.3	45.9	44.5	43.2	41.9
280	58.6	56.7	54.8	53.0	51.3	49.7	48.2	46.7	45.3	43.9	42.7
285	59.7	57.7	55.8	54.0	52.2	50.6	49.0	47.5	46.1	44.7	43.4
290	60.7	58.7	56.8	54.9	53.2	51.5	49.9	48.4	46.9	45.5	44.2
295	61.8	59.7	57.7	55.9	54.1	52.4	50.7	49.2	47.7	46.3	44.9
300	62.8	60.7	58.7	56.8	55.0	53.3	51.6	50.0	48.5	47.1	45.7

Body Mass Index Chart (cont'd.)

5'9"	5'10"	5'11"	6'	6'1"	6'2"	6'3"	6'4"	6'5"	6'6"	6'7"	6'8"
14.8	14.4	14.0	13.6	13.2	12.9	12.5	12.2	11.9	11.6	11.3	11.0
16.3	15.8	15.4	14.9	14.5	14.2	13.8	13.4	13.1	12.7	12.4	12.1
17.8	17.3	16.8	16.3	15.9	15.4	15.0	14.6	14.3	13.9	13.5	13.2
19.2	18.7	18.2	17.7	17.2	16.7	16.3	15.9	15.4	15.1	14.7	14.3
20.7	20.1	19.6	19.0	18.5	18.0	17.5	17.1	16.6	16.2	15.8	15.4
22.2	21.6	21.0	20.4	19.8	19.3	18.8	18.3	17.8	17.4	16.9	16.5
23.7	23.0	22.4	21.7	21.2	20.6	20.0	19.5	19.0	18.5	18.1	17.6
25.2	24.4	23.8	23.1	22.5	21.9	21.3	20.7	20.2	19.7	19.2	18.7
26.6	25.9	25.2	24.5	23.8	23.2	22.5	22.0	21.4	20.8	20.3	19.8
28.1	27.3	26.6	25.8	25.1	24.4	23.8	23.2	22.6	22.0	21.4	20.9
29.6	28.8	28.0	27.2	26.4	25.7	25.1	24.4	23.8	23.2	22.6	22.0
30.3	29.5	28.7	27.9	27.1	26.4	25.7	25.0	24.4	23.7	23.1	22.6
31.1	30.2	29.4	28.5	27.8	27.0	26.3	25.6	25.0	24.3	23.7	23.1
31.8	30.9	30.0	29.2	28.4	27.7	26.9	26.2	25.5	24.9	24.3	23.7
32.6	31.6	30.7	29.9	29.1	28.3	27.6	26.8	26.1	25.5	24.8	24.2
33.3	32.4	31.4	30.6	29.7	28.9	28.2	27.4	26.7	26.1	25.4	24.8
34.0	33.1	32.1	31.3	30.4	29.6	28.8	28.1	27.3	26.6	26.0	25.3
34.8	33.8	32.8	31.9	31.1	30.2	29.4	28.7	27.9	27.2	26.5	25.9
35.5	34.5	33.5	32.6	31.7	30.9	30.1	29.3	28.5	27.8	27.1	26.4
36.3	35.2	34.2	33.3	32.4	31.5	30.7	29.9	29.1	28.4	27.7	27.0
37.0	35.9	34.9	34.0	33.1	32.2	31.3	30.5	29.7	29.0	28.2	27.5
37.7	36.7	35.6	34.7	33.7	32.8	31.9	31.1	30.3	29.5	28.8	28.1
38.5	37.4	36.3	35.3	34.4	33.5	32.6	31.7	30.9	30.1	29.4	28.6
39.2	38.1	37.0	36.0	35.0	34.1	33.2	32.3	31.5	30.7	29.9	29.2
40.0	38.8	37.7	36.7	35.7	34.7	33.8	32.9	32.1	31.3	30.5	29.7
40.7	39.5	38.4	37.4	36.4	35.4	34.4	33.5	32.7	31.8	31.0	30.3
41.4	40.3	39.1	38.1	37.0	36.0	35.0	34.3	33.3	32.4	31.6	30.8
42.2	41.0	39.8	38.7	37.7	36.7	35.7	34.8	33.9	33.0	32.2	31.4
42.9	41.7	40.5	39.4	38.3	37.3	36.3	35.4	34.5	33.6	32.7	31.9
43.7	42.4	41.2	40.1	39.0	38.0	36.9	36.0	35.1	34.2	33.3	32.5
44.4	43.1	41.9	40.8	39.7	38.6	37.6	36.6	35.6	34.7	33.9	33.0

characteristics such as age, sex, and frame size, but others do not. None of the charts make provisions for individuals who have excess muscle but not excess fat (e.g., weight lifters), yet they would be classified as obese according to these charts.

The most accurate way to determine body fat is to weigh people underwater. However, few people have access to the laboratories that have the special equipment for this approach. Therefore, most body fat measurements are done using the skinfold thickness measurement or the bioelectrical impedance analysis (BIA). Both are commonly used in health clubs and commercial weight-loss establishments. During a skinfold test, an examiner uses an instrument called a caliper to measure the thickness of skin and subcutaneous fat at specific sites, usually the back of the upper arm and the abdomen. The BIA sends a harmless electrical current through selected body sites to determine the total percentage of body water. This percentage is used to calculate estimated body fat and lean body mass figures.

Both approaches can give a wide margin of error. To get a general idea of whether you are obese, use this simple technique (you need a ruler and someone to take the measurement). Extend your arm out in front of you with the palm up. Using the forefinger and thumb of your other hand, gently grasp the skin on the underside of your upper arm and pull it away from your body. Ask your partner to measure the thickness of the skin that is between your fingers. If you are between ages 20 and 40, ⅝ inch is "good," ⅞ inch is "average," and 1⅛ inches is "poor." If you are older than 40, ¾ inch is "good," 1 inch is "average," and 1¼ inches is "poor."

Apples and Pears
Are you an apple or a pear? Physicians often use these labels to identify people who carry their weight either around their

waist and abdomen—an "apple"—or around their hips and buttocks—a "pear." Women typically, but not always, are pears, while men usually accumulate a fat buildup around their abdomens. Apples have a higher risk of developing the health problems associated with obesity. To find out whether you are an apple or a pear, determine your waist-to-hip ratio. To do so, you need a measuring tape.

- Measure your waist at its narrowest point, then measure your hips at the widest point.
- Divide the waist measurement by the hip measurement. For example, if your waist is 33 inches and your hips are 45 inches, 33 divided by 45 = 0.74.
- A waist-to-hip ratio of more than 0.80 for women or 1.0 for men identifies an apple.

What Causes Overweight/Obesity?

From a scientific view, obesity occurs when people consume more calories than they burn. What causes this imbalance between the amount of calories consumed and used is unclear; however, it is likely a combination of genetics, environment, emotional-psychological considerations, and medical factors.

Genetics

Some people seem to lack the internal programming that tells the body and mind that there is no danger of starvation. Such genetic misprogramming may be inherited. Researchers believe genes have about a 33 percent stake in determining people's weight. People who are biologically predisposed to being overweight can, and have, successfully lost weight or kept it off in the first place. Other genetic factors include the following:

• In 1994, researchers discovered the obesity (ob) gene in mice. This gene produces the hormone *leptin*. Low levels of leptin may encourage the body to retain fat, but it is still unknown whether the hormone contributes to the regulation of body fat in humans. If it does, scientists believe leptin could prevent weight gain in people prone to obesity.

• The metabolic rate of two people of the same sex, age, and body type may vary as much as 20 percent. The difference in resting metabolic expenditure, or RME, can have a significant effect on body weight because RME accounts for approximately 60 to 75 percent of a person's total daily energy use.

• Black women expend less metabolic energy while at rest (RME) than do white women, and black women lose less weight and gain more weight than do white women when not treated. Overall, black women use 5 percent fewer calories while sitting than white women do, and similar findings have been reported between white men and black and Asian men.

Emotional-Psychological Factors

One common misconception is that weight loss is about willpower; it is *not*. It's about understanding the factors that cause you to overeat or to continue with habits that contribute to being overweight. Once you understand your relationship with food, you can understand why you eat when you're not hungry. We look at these issues in Chapter 8.

Environmental-Cultural Factors

• **Eating Habits.** In today's stressful society, many people eat on the run, which often means buying high-fat, high-calorie fast food; snacking on candy, cookies, and other treats in the office during the day; tossing a prepackaged, chemical-laden dinner into the microwave; or grabbing a late meal and then falling asleep in front of the television.

• **Cultural, Familial, and Social Factors.** For example,

families for whom fried foods, heavy sauces, or sweets are routine fare are indoctrinating their children to food preferences they will likely find difficult to change. Being ordered as a child to clean off your plate may develop into overeating habits as an adult.

Medical and Drug-Related Factors

Experts estimate that 1 percent of people who are overweight can attribute it, at least partly, to a disease or to medication. Many health practitioners, however, believe there are medical factors other than the few diseases mentioned below that affect people's ability to lose weight. These conditions are usually overlooked by conventional physicians but are often part of the routine examination done by naturopaths. These factors, listed below, are key for many people who struggle between a healthy weight and being overweight.

• **Disease.** Hypothyroidism is the most common in this category. If the thyroid gland malfunctions, the metabolism rate may slow down greatly. Less common medical conditions that can cause obesity include Cushing's syndrome and neurological problems that can lead to overeating.

• **Chronic Yeast Infection.** This condition is caused by an imbalance in the body of a yeast fungus called *Candida albicans*. It contributes to weight gain by making the body store unwanted fat, especially among both young and postmenopausal women.

• **Enzyme Imbalance.** Enzymes help convert foods into nutrients the body can use in order to digest food and initiate metabolic activity. Enzyme deficiencies can cause insufficient absorption of food and food cravings.

• **Sluggish Lymphatic System.** The lymphatic system eliminates cellular waste and environmental poisons from the body and plays a major role in fat metabolism. If you eat too much fat, the system can become congested and cause cellulite, tissue swelling, and a slowdown in your metabolic rate.

• **Toxic Liver.** The liver detoxifies the blood, manages nutrients and hormones, and metabolizes fats, all of which make it a vital part of weight management and maintenance. Many people overburden the liver with a poor diet and high stress, which often leaves the liver in a toxic state.

• **Food Allergies and Intolerances.** Food allergies and intolerance are overlooked contributors to overweight, binge eating, compulsive eating, and food cravings. It is estimated that 2 percent of the population have food allergies and that at least 40 percent have food intolerance. Chronic symptoms such as weight gain, arthritis, and gastritis are common among people with food intolerance.

• **Insulin Resistance.** Some people's cells resist the effort of insulin to penetrate them, so the extra insulin builds up in the bloodstream and causes the insulin level to increase. Insulin resistance may stimulate the appetite and increase the amount of fat the body stores. Researchers believe about 25 percent of people are insulin resistant.

Drug-Related Obesity

Certain drugs can cause weight gain by increasing appetite, promoting fluid retention, and stimulating hormones that cause weight gain, or by unknown mechanisms (see the table below). Most drugs associated with weight gain fall into the latter category. Although these drugs are not the primary reason for weight gain, they can play a significant contributing role and so deserve mention.

DRUG-INDUCED WEIGHT GAIN

Drugs that Stimulate the Appetite: corticosteroids (e.g., beclomethasone, betamethasone, prednisone), estrogens, and antidepressants (e.g., amitriptyline, desipramine, doxepin, nortriptyline, and venlafaxine)

Drugs that Cause Water Retention: Antihypertensive drugs, including certain calcium channel blockers and beta-blockers; also estrogens and corticosteroids

Drugs that Cause Weight Gain Indirectly: Ironically, oral hypoglycemic agents, which are used to treat adult-onset diabetes, stimulate weight gain in the very population that usually needs to lose weight.

Drugs that Cause Weight Gain by Unknown Mechanisms: antihistamines (including methyldopa, clonidine, guanadrel sulfate, lithium, thioridazine, and alprazolam)

Obesity: How Unhealthy Is It?

Why do you want to lose weight? If you are like most people who are overweight, it's because you want to look better and feel better about yourself, and/or you want to improve your health. Both reasons go hand in hand: when your health improves, you feel better physically, emotionally, and spiritually. Conversely, bonuses come with weight loss: a significantly decreased risk of troublesome and sometimes fatal diseases; and increased energy, better mood, and improved self-esteem.

Obesity carries high health and economic price tags. For example, if you are obese:

• You have a 3.8 greater risk of developing NIDDM (also known as Type II diabetes).

• Your chances of developing high blood pressure are double that of normal-weight individuals. Hypertension affects about 26 percent of people who are obese.

• You have an increased risk of developing breast cancer and colon cancer.

• You have a 2.1 times greater risk of getting hypercholesterolemia (high cholesterol levels), a significant factor in stroke, heart disease, and circulatory problems, if you are aged 20 to 44.

Some researchers question the validity of these statistics, and research into the role of exercise, genetics, and environmental factors in obesity continues. In most cases, however, it appears that being overweight carries certain health risks, and that being 30 percent or more over ideal body weight is a definite health hazard.

Are You at Risk for Health Complications?

Doctors generally agree that people who are 20 percent or more overweight can gain significant health benefits (i.e., lower blood pressure and cholesterol levels) from as little as a 10- to 20-pound weight loss. Individuals who are more than 20 percent overweight run an especially high risk of health problems if any of the following factors are true for them:

• A family history of diabetes or heart disease. People with close relatives who have had these medical conditions are more likely also to develop these problems if they are obese.

• Presence of high blood pressure, high cholesterol levels, and high blood sugar levels, which are all warning signs of some obesity-associated diseases.

• "Apple" shape. People who carry their extra weight in the abdominal area may be at greater risk of heart disease, diabetes, or cancer than people of the same weight who carry their extra weight in the hip and buttocks (pear-shaped).

Below we look at the physical and psychological health risks associated with being overweight.

• **Cardiovascular Diseases.** Diseases in this category are the leading cause of death in the United States. Nearly 70 percent of cases diagnosed as cardiovascular disease are related to obesity. The most common problems include hypertension, atherosclerosis (also called hardening of the arteries), coronary heart disease, congestive heart failure, and angina. People who are severely overweight are believed to be at significantly higher risk of developing these diseases.

• **Diabetes.** Type II diabetes (noninsulin-dependent diabetes mellitus, or NIDDM) is five times more common among people who are obese. According to the National Institute of Diabetes and Digestive and Kidney Disease, nearly 80 percent of people with noninsulin-dependent diabetes (NIDDM) are obese. Both NIDDM and stroke contribute to an increase in obesity-related deaths.

• **Cancer.** A link between obesity and cancer was first documented in the 1940s. Since that time, a growing number of studies suggest an association between obesity and cancer of the colon, rectum, and prostate among men and of the cervix, ovary, breast, endometrium, and gallbladder among women. The American Cancer Society has also found higher rates of stomach, uterine, and kidney cancer among obese individuals. The society also notes that an estimated "one-third of the annual 500,000 deaths from cancer in the United States, including the most common sites such as breast, colon, and prostate, may be attributed to undesirable dietary practices."

• **Musculoskeletal Problems.** Excess weight often causes arthritis, especially osteoarthritis, and other painful joint conditions. The joints most often affected include the hips, knees, spine, and ankles. Foot pain is also associated with obesity. People who are overweight typically develop osteo-porosis at an earlier age and have a more debilitating form of the disease. Weight loss can help prevent onset of this disorder and significantly reduce the pain, swelling, and disability once the damage has been established.

• **Reproductive Disorders.** Severely obese women have more problems with ovulation than do women of normal weight, and frequently also have raised levels of male sex hormones. This combination causes fertility problems, and weight loss often is the only approach needed to restore fertility. The incidence of cesarean births and spontaneous abortion is higher among obese women. Obesity among men is often linked with impotence and low sperm count.

• **Gallbladder Disease.** Obesity and high intake of fat are both risk factors for the formation of stones in the gallbladder. Gallstones are usually made of cholesterol and form when the amount of cholesterol in the bile exceeds the organ's ability to eliminate it.

• **Other Physical Weight-Related Problems.** *Sleep apnea* refers to episodes of stopped breathing, or apnea, while sleeping, that last longer than ten seconds. The majority of the 20 million Americans who suffer from some degree of sleep apnea are overweight. *Gout* is a type of arthritis in which there is an excess of uric acid in the joint linings. A combination of excess weight and consumption of foods high in purines (red meat, liver, cheese), which break down into uric acid, lead to the formation of crystals that settle in the extremities and develop into gout. *Varicose veins* are the prominent blue lines, sometimes painful, that form in the legs when the valves in the leg veins are stretched and damaged because of excessive weight and pressure.

• **Psychological and Emotional Hazards.** Both men and women equate beauty and success with being thin, and pressure is especially great on women to be slender. Says Susie Orbach, author of *Fat Is a Feminist Issue:* ''Women absorb a powerfully contradictory message vis-à-vis food and eating. It is good for others, but bad for the woman herself; healthy for others, harmful to the woman herself; full of love and nurturance for others, full of self-indulgence for herself.'' To further support this misguided concept, Louis Aronne, M.D., author of _Weigh Less, Live Longer,_ found that ''most of the country's male business leaders are above-average weight yet most of their wives weigh less than the norm.'' These are but two examples of society's misguided standards.

Other psychological factors associated with overweight include a distorted body image and attitude about food and weight; feeling self-conscious about eating in front of other people; depression and feelings of failure and hopelessness when fad diets don't work; and lack of sufficient encouragement and assistance from physicians, family, and friends.

Social prejudice is another consequence of obesity and often manifests as job discrimination and feelings of alienation in social settings. Overweight children and teens in particular often suffer ridicule at the hands of their peers, making it difficult or impossible for them to join in play groups, sporting events, and dating.

In this chapter you read about how your body works with you and against you in your quest to lose weight. You learned about the many factors that may be involved in your being overweight and some of the medical conditions associated with obesity. What you've learned can be used to help you lose that weight.

A successful weight loss and maintenance program requires a lifelong commitment—to health, well-being, vitality, and feeling good about yourself. This book talks about how to achieve that commitment using safe, natural approaches. Unfortunately, many people are drawn to fad diets and prescription and over-the-counter drugs only to discover, sooner or later, that the ''magic'' potion doesn't work as promised or, worse, that it has caused health problems. In Chapter 2 we look at some of the popular diet programs, weight loss drugs, and dietary food aids available on the market and at the pros and cons of their use.

CHAPTER TWO

The Problem with Fad Diets and Diet Drugs

"Lose 30 Pounds in 3 Days." "Eat All the Chocolate You Want and Still Lose Weight." "Magic Pill Sheds Pounds Without Dieting." You've seen and heard the promises and the "virtues" of scores of fad diet plans, weight loss pills, diet foods, and weight loss centers. Most of them make fantastic though unsubstantiated claims, yet they have accomplished their goal if they draw you in with your money in hand. Some weight loss programs are based on sound nutritional research that emphasizes wholesome food and exercise, but the prices you pay for the program's "special" foods and program support is often excessive, and the success rate claimed by such programs is frequently exaggerated or misleading. Diet pills and diet foods claiming to melt away fat or take away your appetite may also be taking away your health.

In this chapter we look at the pros and cons of some of the high-priced diet programs, fad diets, weight loss products, and weight loss drugs currently in the marketplace. After reading this section you'll probably be ready to say, "There's got to be a better way," and there is. In the next seven chapters we present a view of the natural medicine approaches to weight loss and how you can use them to make your quest for a lighter, more energetic you a reality.

Fasting and Skipping Meals

Although you may think fasting is a quick way to lose weight, it generally is not a good way to use this healing technique, and for several reasons.

One is that fasting provides only temporary results because much of the weight you lose will be water weight. Two, it can stimulate a tendency to overeat when you come off the fast, which defeats the purpose. Three, it does not allow you to establish good eating habits and develop healthy food choices.

Fasting may be beneficial for some people who have a weight problem. Some health professionals, for example, believe that with proper supervision and a firm commitment to adopt healthy eating habits, overweight people can use a short five- to ten-day fast to motivate them toward making dietary changes. Such fasts should be followed immediately by a healthy eating plan and exercise program. Fasting also may be helpful for people who have allergies to foods that contribute to their being overweight. (See Chapter 3 for healthy eating plans and information about food allergies.)

Individuals who fast for a week or more risk losing essential lean body mass and fluids and are in danger of muscle wasting, liver and kidney damage, and gout. In cases of extreme obesity, some people undergo medically supervised water-only fasts for up to thirty days. Such attempts are done in the hospital and are rigorously controlled. Fasting is not recommended if you have any of the following conditions: fatigue, low immunity, low blood pressure, heart problems, cancer, peptic ulcers, or nutritional deficiencies, or if you are pregnant, nursing, or preparing for surgery.

Skipping meals, especially breakfast, is a popular strategy among dieters. Too often this weight loss effort backfires as people are ravenous by nighttime and make up for the unconsumed calories by eating a big dinner and snacks. In fact, skipping breakfast is not a good idea for several reasons, but of special interest to people who are trying to lose weight is that not eating breakfast can reduce your metabolic rate by 4 to 5 percent, while eating raises metabolism. It is also best to eat when you will be the most active, and for most people that is the morning and afternoon rather than after dinner. Rather than skip meals, C. Wayne Callaway, M.D., associate professor of medicine at George Washington University, recommends that people eat at least 50 percent of their calories by the end of lunch. This not only gives your body a fighting chance to burn the calories off, it also keeps your energy level high.

Yo-Yo Dieting

Repeated attempts to lose weight, and the subsequent regain of the same amount of weight or more, is known as *weight cycling,* or *yo-yo dieting.* Although this is a common phenomenon, thus far researchers have had little success in drawing firm conclusions about the health aspects of yo-yo dieting. Some significant information has been gathered from the Framingham Heart Study (a study of heart disease that began in 1948 and has included more than 5,000 men and women), which suggests that weight cycling is associated with higher rates of death and coronary heart disease.

According to Robert B. Baron, M.D., of the University of California San Francisco, Division of General Internal Medicine, animal and human studies of weight cycling indicate many possible adverse effects, including: further weight loss being more difficult; increase in total body fat and central obesity; increase in blood cholesterol and triglyceride levels;

increase in insulin resistance; rise in blood pressure; increase in food efficiency (it takes less food for the body to operate efficiently); decrease in energy expenditure (muscle uses more calories than fat does); and increase in fat and liver enzymes.

One reason yo-yo dieting may directly cause weight gain is that it appears to damage permanently the ability of brown fat to respond to norepinephrine, which causes the level of thermogenesis to decrease. A reduced thermogenesis level discourages the body from burning fat and increases appetite.

While the debate continues about the negative effects of yo-yo dieting, researchers do understand much more about how metabolism is affected during weight loss.

Popular Diets: Or, How to Waste Time and Money and Risk Your Health

Though this is a book on natural weight loss options, there are various other diet plans that deserve quick mention because many of them involve potential health risks and are designed to make you lighter in the wallet and often nowhere else. We discuss some of the general categories below.

High-Protein Diets

High-protein, low-carbohydrate diets have been around for decades. Some of the early ones included the Stillman Diet, Dr. Atkins' Diet, and the Scarsdale Diet. These eating plans were shown to cause many medical problems, including a sometimes dramatic increase in cholesterol levels. Some people on these diets developed ketosis, in which the body lacks sufficient carbohydrates and thus breaks down fat faster than it can rid itself of the "refuse," or ketones. These ketones cause weakness, nausea, and constipation and may lead to kidney problems. Your body draws water from your tissues and the water will remove the ketones. This results in dehydration and the resulting weight loss you experience is actually from water.

Slightly modified high-protein diets (the most recent "allow" 40 percent of calories from carbohydrates, a bit higher than earlier plans) are still with us today. These include *Dr. Atkins' New Diet Revolution,* Barry Sears's *The Zone,* Cliff Sheats's *Lean Bodies Total Fitness,* Adele Puhn's *The 5-Day Miracle Diet,* and Michael and Mary Dan Eades's *Protein Power.* Like their predecessors, these diet plans are "science fiction," says Alice Lichtenstein, a researcher at the Jean Mayer U.S. Department of Agriculture Human Nutrition Research Center on Aging at Tufts University in Boston. The most vocal of the high-protein diet advocates make money not only off the books they write but also on the diet products they sell. Two examples are Cliff Sheats, who promotes dietary supplements and his own brand of beef, and Barry Sears, who peddles nutrition bars.

The claims of high-protein diet gurus have not been backed up by controlled, scientific studies. Some of the statements made by these individuals include the following:

• Claim: *Americans are fatter because they are eating less fat.* In fact, the National Center for Health Statistics reports that the average American ate 81.4 grams of fat a day in the late 1970s and 82 grams per day in the late 1980s. In addition, Americans are eating 100 to 300 more calories per day, and exercising less, than they were in the 1970s. Thus, not only hasn't fat consumption decreased; caloric intake has risen and exercise has fallen. These are far more persuasive reasons why Americans are getting heavier.

• Claim: *Carbohydrates cause obesity.* The return of high-protein diets is based largely on the myth that carbohydrates and insulin work together to cause weight gain. Many authors of books on high-protein diets claim that eating carbohydrates triggers the secretion of insulin, which in turn signals the carbohydrates to be stored as fat rather than be used as energy. These claims are unsubstantiated. In fact, all calories, regardless of their source, are converted into glucose to be used for energy. The only time glucose is stored as fat is when an excess number of calories are consumed and not burned, be they 3,000 calories from chocolate eclairs or carrots.

Experts who have evaluated low-carbohydrate, high-protein plans say the only reason people can lose weight on them is that they will eat fewer calories, not because of the claims made by the authors. High-protein diets are known for their ability to cause quick weight loss, but most of the initial loss is water rather than fat. More important, however, is that these diets are not nutritionally sound. Many high-protein foods, such as meats and cheese, are also high in saturated fat and extremely low in fiber. People on high-protein diets tend to be deficient in vitamins and minerals because they do not consume the necessary vegetables, legumes, fruits, and grains. Numerous scientific studies show that fiber and vegetables are instrumental in preventing disease, that high protein intake is the cause of osteoporosis (and not insufficient calcium intake, as many mistakenly believe) and leads to kidney stones, and that carbohydrates are essential for energy.

Single-Food Diets

Certainly doomed for failure is any diet that focuses on a single food or food group or severely limits the types of food you can eat each day. Some of them include the Popcorn Diet, the Grapefruit Diet, and the Cabbage Soup Diet. You will probably experience some quick weight loss, but it will return once you stop this artificial way of eating and return to normal consumption. Such diet plans also often cause side effects, such as headache, diarrhea, constipation, and gastric upset, as well as vitamin and mineral deficiencies.

The Cabbage Soup Diet is reportedly "recommended" by physicians for patients who are preparing for heart surgery. Promotions for this plan claim you can lose 10 to 17 pounds in just seven days if you consume unlimited amounts of cabbage soup and other selected foods on certain days. Although the soup itself is packed with vitamins and minerals, it does not provide other essential nutrients, and it certainly does not contain a magic ingredient to make you lose weight. Weight loss occurs because of reduced caloric intake and fluid loss.

The Grapefruit Diet, which first surfaced in the 1930s as the Hollywood Diet, has undergone many variations over the decades. It calls for eating a few select vegetables, small amounts of protein, and grapefruit, which are said to contain a special fat-burning enzyme. Not only is this diet deficient in nutrients; it also is less than 800 calories per day.

Food-Combining Diets

In the 1930s, author William H. Hay introduced the idea that starches and proteins should be eaten separately, and that fruits should not be eaten with either starches or proteins. A variation on that theme appeared in 1981, when Judy Mazel unveiled the Beverly Hills Diet, in which she claimed that fruit enzymes could burn up calories before they turned to fat and that you should eat proteins and carbohydrates at different times. This diet was called "the worst entry in the diet-fad derby" by the *Journal of the American Medical Association.* The diet is low in protein, iron, niacin, calcium, and other vital nutrients. Much of the weight loss associated with this diet is the result of the diarrhea it causes.

Four years later, Marilyn Diamond wrote *Fit for Life,* in which she advocated eating only fruit and fruit juice before noon and other specific food combinations throughout the day. However, there is no scientific evidence that the body processes specific food combinations any differently than random ones. Thus you are wasting your time and potentially risking your health if you decide to follow a food-combining diet plan.

Very Low Calorie Diets (VLCDs)

These plans typically consist of consumption of a high-protein food product, such as liquid protein, for a total of 400 to 800 calories per day for a maximum of thirty days. Such diets are usually used by severely obese individuals who are trying to lose 50 or more pounds, and should only be done under direct medical supervision. When handled in this way, many physicians believe VLCDs are safe, even though there are several problems with them.

One common adverse effect is the formation of gallstones; another is the high cost of the liquid protein formula, which limits its use to people of higher economic means. Many obesity experts also warn that placing people on liquid protein diets is artificial and does not help them develop proper eating habits and attitudes about food. Once they stop the VLCD, they usually revert back to their old eating patterns and regain the weight they lost.

One reason VLCDs can be successful, but only in the short run, is that once you reduce your caloric intake, it takes approximately three months of consuming the same number of calories before your metabolism levels off and you will no longer lose weight at that calorie level. Use of VLCDs for up to thirty days can help severely obese individuals get a "jump start" on weight loss, but longer use can be dangerous to your health. Overall, the key is still to keep caloric intake up by eating your recommended caloric intake and by having a good exercise program.

Diet Programs

Every year, about 8 million Americans plop down their money on one or more of the ten thousand–plus commercial weight-loss programs in operation. And what do they get for their hard-earned dollars? Not great results, according to the NIH. Although many of the programs talk about the importance of a long-range maintenance program, the words fall on deaf ears. About 95 percent of those who enroll in organized weight-loss programs regain two-thirds of the lost poundage within one to three years.

Commercial diet programs such as Weight Watchers, Jenny Craig, Nutri/System, The Diet Center, and dozens of others listed in the Yellow Pages of your telephone book make a variety of claims targeted at people who are desperate to lose weight. Throughout the 1990s, the Federal Trade Commission (FTC) reached agreements with several large weight-loss programs regarding their advertising. Jenny Craig, for example, agreed to stop deceptive advertising and provide more complete information on the health risks, pricing schemes, and actual success rates associated with their programs. No weight loss company can guarantee that participants will be able to keep the weight off after the program ends. But often you must look closely or quickly for the tiny type that says "Results not typical" at the bottom of print ads or that flashes across the television screen.

Nor can a weight loss company claim that its plan will keep weight off permanently. While many companies claim they do not keep data on how many of their clients keep the weight off for one year or longer, skeptics of that claim believe that not only are the statistics kept, but because they are so unfavorable they are simply not reported. Based on the high failure rate noted by the NIH, such secrecy would not be surprising.

The FTC also requires that consumers be informed about

any additional costs associated with an advertised weight-loss program, such as special prepackaged foods or supplements they are expected to purchase. These items mean big money to program operators and to the salespeople who sell them on commission, which can be as high as 50 percent of their income. Consumers get very costly food that adds up to about 1,200 calories a day—where they could get similar food for a fraction of the cost at any supermarket.

Overall, commercial weight-loss programs seem to offer some form of temporary structure and hope for many overweight individuals. The key word here is *temporary*. The high dropout rate for many commercial weight-loss programs can be traced to the rigidity of some programs, the unrealistic weight goals set for participants in many programs, and the often high cost.

"Wonder" Diet Drugs and Diet Aids

The ultimate dream of all overweight people is to find a pill or a food that will magically melt away fat, let them eat as much as they want without gaining weight, or let them lose weight without effort. And though most know that such products do not exist, they still buy millions of dollars' worth of diet foods and aids that make these claims. In this section we look at some of these items.

Of all the "magic" diet drugs on the market, two captured the spotlight for a time: dexfenfluramine (Redux), approved by the FDA in June 1996 and withdrawn by the manufacturer in 1997; and the combination phen-fen (phentermine and fenfluramine), which individually received FDA approval for use in weight loss but not as a compound. Fenfluramine was subsequently withdrawn from the market by the manufacturer in 1997; phentermine remains available for weight loss.

Redux: What Went Wrong

Redux had been studied since the 1960s, and by 1997 reviews of its long-term use showed that people who took the drug for one year did not lose significantly more weight than people who took a placebo. In fact, people who took the drug lost only an average of 5.5 pounds more than people who took a placebo. Along with the few extra pounds they shed, many of those who took Redux also experienced drowsiness, headaches, dizziness, anxiety, and sleep difficulties. A more serious risk associated with taking Redux is that of primary pulmonary hypertension, a rare and often fatal disease usually seen in women aged 30 to 50 years. The disease causes fluid to build up in the lungs as a result of high blood pressure in the veins and arteries. In a study that compared people with pulmonary hypertension to healthy people, those with the disease were twenty-three times more likely to have taken dexfenfluramine for weight loss.

The Fury over Phen-Fen

The phen-fen bandwagon had no problem attracting riders. In 1996, 18 million prescriptions were written for this combination of a Prozac-like drug that creates satiety and calm by increasing the level of serotonin in the brain (fenfluramine) and an amphetamine-like stimulant (phentermine). It also produces side effects, including sleeplessness, depression, and headaches. Most doctors agree it should be administered only to individuals who are at least 20 to 30 percent overweight. Wyeth-Ayerst Laboratories, Inc., makers of fenfluramine, warned physicians that taking the drug with phentermine is "not recommended," and the combination was banned in Sweden. In July 1997, the Food and Drug Administration (FDA) and Mayo Clinic announced that phen-fen may cause heart valve deformities and irreversible lung damage.

The final blow to the combination drug was delivered in

September 1997 when the FDA asked the manufacturers of fenfluramine and Redux (see above) to pull their products from the market. About 100 cases of a very rare valve disease had been found among people taking phen-fen, fenfluramine alone, or Redux alone. In addition, the FDA had conducted echocardiograms on nearly 300 patients who were taking the combination or Redux alone and discovered that 30 percent of them had abnormalities, a much higher rate than expected. Though the other half of the phen-fen combination, phentermine, was not removed from the marketplace, the recall caused many of the more than 6 million users of phen-fen to go cold turkey or find alternatives. (See Herbal Forms of Phen-Fen in Chapter 6.)

Phenylpropanolamine

A third diet drug deserves mention because not only has it been available longer than either of the above-mentioned newer drugs, it is available over the counter. Phenylpropanolamine, or PPA, is an appetite suppressant and a stimulant that is found in brand-name diet aids such as Dexatrim, Appedrine, Mini Slim, and Acutrim. The American Medical Association's drug evaluations team lists PPA as being "minimally effective," while the FDA's advisory review panel admits that they approved the drug based on inaccurate studies.

Despite these facts, Americans consume 6 billion doses of products a year that contain PPA, while 95 percent of developed nations in the world have already banned the drug. Adverse effects include increased blood pressure, headache, nausea, nervousness, anxiety, seizures, irritability, and loss of concentration. The drug's easy accessibility to teenagers has made it popular with young people, who abuse it in their desire to lose weight.

Diet Food Aids

If you believe the advertisements, you could eat yourself slim and trim with the many dietary food aids on the market. One problem is, they really are not offering you anything that you couldn't do on your own . . . and without the high cost. Another is that they are a temporary solution. These products are designed for quick weight loss rather than a lifelong, healthy eating program. Their use often throws people into a yo-yo dieting pattern that has them going back for more products or just giving up altogether and regaining any weight they lost.

Products and programs that provide fewer than 800 calories per day are potentially quite dangerous and should be avoided. A variant on this concept is Ultra Slim-Fast, which instructs users to drink two shakes per day (about 200 calories each) and eat a nutritious 400- to 600-calorie dinner. Although the shakes do provide adequate levels of protein, vitamins, and minerals, users typically lose some weight quickly only to regain it once they go off the routine. Diet plans that require people to eat or drink specific products in lieu of a meal on a daily basis quickly lose their appeal because they are not plans people would want to follow for the rest of their life.

You also need to be aware of misleading or inaccurate information that accompanies these products. The Herbalife Slim and Trim weight control program, for example, has a protein food that the label claims "is scientifically formulated to satisfy your hunger and help reduce nervousness and irritability, which often comes when restricting food intake. It burns fat and builds muscle." You are led to believe that this protein formula will burn fat while it builds muscle, but the truth is that protein does not burn fat. Nor does it reduce nervous irritability. Another fact is that a diet high in protein can be nauseating, which is not the optimal way to reduce your appetite! Yet another problem with these and other weight loss food aids is that people are not instructed on how to eat once they lose the weight.

Dying to Be Thin

For some individuals, the desire to be thin becomes an obsession. This intense desire is usually fueled by various factors, such as emotional and personality problems, family and peer pressures, societal pressures, and possibly genetic susceptibility. Of the two most common eating disorders, bulimia nervosa is practiced by more people. It involves a cycle of bingeing on large amounts of food and then purging by vomiting or using laxatives, diuretics, diet pills, or enemas. The second type, anorexia nervosa, is a state of starvation and emaciation that is usually accomplished by little or no food consumption and sometimes accompanied by purging. People who are anorexic lose between 15 and 60 percent of their normal body weight.

Estimates of both anorexia and bulimia in the United States range from 2 to 18 percent. About 90 percent are women, although the 10 percent attributed to men may be higher because men are more likely to conceal an eating disorder than women are.

Both anorexia and bulimia can cause numerous health problems, including digestive disorders, arrhythmia, muscle loss, weakness and fatigue, and even death.

The lure to "be thin, be successful, be popular" is indeed enticing, yet deciding to lose weight using "magic" pills or formulas, crash diets, unhealthy eating habits, or fasting is not the answer. You've already seen that losing weight is not a matter of just reducing caloric intake and exercising. Many factors, some of them subtle, can have an adverse effect on your ability to lose weight.

But enough talk. In the next seven chapters you will read

about how various natural techniques, supplements, and other helpful aids can facilitate your weight loss efforts. Depending on the remedy we're talking about, you'll learn how much to take, how much to do, or where to go to get it. You'll also discover how they work, why they work, and even why they may not always work. Curious? Let's go!

PART TWO

HEALTHY, HOLISTIC WEIGHT LOSS

Welcome to a world of natural, healthy weight loss. This section contains two categories of weight loss techniques: (1) the mainstays of any successful weight loss plan—a high-fiber, lower-fat eating plan and an exercise program, complete with suggestions to get you on your way immediately; and (2) holistic complementary remedies and methods to help you reach your weight goals. Before you start on your new path to a lighter, healthier you, we recommend you have a complete physical examination and consultation with your physician, naturopath, or other health care provider who is knowledgeable about nutrition and weight loss. Depending on which natural approaches you choose to try, you also may want to consult with a herbalist, yoga instructor, massage therapist, or other holistic health specialists. See Chapter 11 and Appendix A for help in choosing and locating the appropriate experts for your needs.

It is hard to pick up a newspaper or magazine or to watch television without seeing advertisements for weight loss programs, diet pills, fat-dissolving supplements, or other "magic" substances that melt away fat and inches with little or no effort on your part. If these claims were all they purport to be, the following statistic would not be true: Only about 10 percent of obese people permanently shed the pounds and the label of obesity. The fact is, losing weight does take effort, patience, and dedication. In the next few chapters, we offer you approaches that work with your body instead of against it, as many drugs do. We suggest you read Chapter 3 and plan a new food strategy. Then read Chapters 5, 6, 7, and 8 and choose one or more natural approaches that can complement your weight loss efforts. Don't forget Chapter 9; and remember to make it fun! Now you're off—and soon so will be the weight!

CHAPTER THREE

Food Plans: No Fads, No Gimmicks

If you are like most Americans, you have been conditioned to eat an unhealthy diet loaded with fats and cholesterol in the form of meat, fowl, fried foods, dairy products, and lots of processed foods loaded with sugar, preservatives, and chemicals with names too long to pronounce. This way of eating, called the Standard American Diet (or SAD, appropriately named), is usually seriously lacking in fiber and nutrients and contributes to and causes obesity, diabetes, heart disease, high blood pressure, chronic constipation, gallbladder disease, arthritis, osteoporosis, high cholesterol, and various cancers. Quite a sad list.

When you follow the Healthy Eating Lifelong Plan, or HELP, discussed in this chapter, you can lose weight and keep it off, and reverse or significantly reduce the risk of these health problems. Such an eating plan consists of vegetables, fruits, whole grains, beans, and legumes prepared in delicious, low-calorie ways. It provides a nutritious balance of protein, carbohydrates, fat, vitamins, minerals, and fiber. In the pages that follow, we focus on these foods and how they can help you lose weight and keep it off.

You may have tried various diets you've read about in books or magazines. Most of them claim to be "the one" that will make you thinner and keep the pounds off forever. So before you read any further, let us dispel this misconception. **Not Every BODY is the same, so no single diet will work for everyone. Beware of any diet plan that claims it will work for EVERYONE.** There are, however, *general guidelines* that have been shown repeatedly to work for nearly everyone, barring individuals with special or serious medical conditions. It is those guidelines we offer to you in this chapter. In most cases, if you follow the food suggestions and complement them with exercise and natural options in this book, you will lose weight and keep it off.

First, however, let's take a brief look at the phenomenon known as "dieting" and the relationship between you and your food. A better understanding of these issues can make following the guidelines . . . well, a piece of cake!

Dieting Can Make You Fatter

You've decided to go on a diet. Say you've been consuming 2,200 calories a day; you reduce your intake to 1,000 calories a day. You lose weight, at least initially. Then, after several weeks on this severely restricted plan, you stop losing. All along you've been hungry and weak and now you're discouraged. When you return to your old eating habits, you gain back the weight you lost, and, if you are like most dieters, a few extra pounds. Dieting has made you fatter.

You are not alone: most dieters who resort to calorie counting and food deprivation—and the majority of dieters try this approach at least once—end up just as heavy or heavier than they were before the diet. But why does dieting make you fatter?

Whenever you drastically limit the amount of calories you consume, the body switches into "survival mode." This built-in mechanism has kept our species alive in lean times. It still operates that way for people in regions where food is in short supply. But for people who want to lose weight, survival mode may seem to conspire against them. Here's how it works.

Two mechanisms at work in weight control are metabolic rate and set point. **Metabolic rate** is the speed at which the body releases energy from the food consumed and uses that energy to function. When you don't give the body enough calories (energy) to run optimally, it responds by reducing the amount of energy it needs to survive and maintain the **set point:** a weight the body tries to maintain despite attempts to reduce it.

You can change your set point; however, it takes time for the body to readjust to a point that will not sabotage the attempt to lose weight. That's why a successful shift in set point requires patience along with HELP, regular exercise, and mind-body awareness techniques, which are discussed in Chapter 8.

One situation many dieters get into is a repeat cycle of losing and gaining weight, which is called **yo-yo dieting.** Once you are caught in this cycle, each time you try to lose weight you lose more muscle and gain back more fat-storing enzymes, making it increasingly difficult to lose weight permanently. Use of HELP, along with other holistic weight-loss approaches that interest you in this book, prevent you from falling victim to yo-yo dieting.

Hunger Begins in the Brain

The mind-body relationship is key to permanent weight loss. One example of the mind-body link is that between your stomach and your brain. Your stomach may grumble, but hunger really begins in a region of the brain called the *hypo-thalamus.* This appetite and hunger control center dispatches *neurotransmitters,* chemicals that tell you when, what, and how much to eat. When your hypothalamus sends out a surge of neuropeptide Y, for example, you will want carbohydrates. Once you satisfy that urge, the hypothalamus sends out another hormone—serotonin—that says you've had enough.

This message exchange can be easily disturbed. If you greatly reduce your caloric intake or skip meals; if you are under a great deal of stress; or if you are taking drugs that affect brain chemistry, including antidepressants, you may upset the release of serotonin and you won't know when you are full. Low levels of serotonin also may be linked with cravings for sweets. (See Chapter 4, under The Addiction Process.)

A Few Words on Calories

Before you can build your own HELP, you need to set your weight goal and determine how many calories you can consume to meet that goal. Here's a quick way to see what that number is for you. This information is based on more than six years of studies conducted at Rockefeller University by some of the nation's top experts on obesity. The numbers given are for sedentary people; the actual number you may need can be a bit more or less, depending on your level of activity. Use the number you come up with as a guide only; you don't need to count every calorie you eat. In fact, please don't! After a few days or weeks of following HELP, you will sense what foods and amounts are right for you.

Refer to the chart and find the number of calories you need to maintain your current weight by locating the intersection of your height and your weight. We will use LeeAnn as an example. LeeAnn is five feet two inches (62 inches) and weighs 160 pounds. According to the chart, her maintenance calorie need is 2,368 calories (round to nearest hundred, or 2,400).

The healthy, effective way to lose weight is to do so slowly. Suddenly reducing your caloric intake from 2,400 to 1,200, for example, is difficult for most people to do. Many obesity experts recommend you set realistic, workable goals for yourself—say, each goal is to lose 10 percent of your body weight. This approach reduces the chance that you'll become discouraged and quit. Let's look at LeeAnn again.

LeeAnn wants to lose at least 30 pounds. Her first goal is to lose 10 percent of her body weight, or 16 pounds. To determine how many calories she should consume to reach that goal, she multiplies 2,400 by 0.75, which equals 1,800 calories. She will consume approximately 1,800 calories a day until she reaches her first goal of 144 pounds. Then she should give her body time to readjust her metabolism and set point (see page 41) for a minimum of one month. Her next goal is another 10 percent (16 pounds more). To determine her new calorie requirement, she multiplies 2,400 by 0.65 and gets 1,560 calories. If she chooses to lose another 10 percent, she would multiply 2,400 by 0.55 for 1,320 calories.

Building a Healthy Weight-Loss/Maintenance Food Program

You can create your own HELP with the suggestions we discuss below. The program you build needs to satisfy you physically, psychologically, and emotionally or else you won't follow it. The guidelines in this chapter can certainly fulfill the physical part; help with the psychological and emotional portions can be found in subsequent chapters.

Forget the diet mentality of deprivation, boredom, and suffering. You can take positive steps to add vitality and well-being to your life as you subtract pounds. Before you start your new program, get a small notebook and write down everything you eat and drink—meals and snacks—for one

The Calories You Need

Height inches	58	59	60	61	62	63	64	65	66	67	68
Weight lb											
100	1848	1871	1894	1917	1939	1962	1985	2007	2029	2052	2074
105	1887	1910	1934	1957	1980	2003	2026	2049	2072	2095	2117
110	1924	1948	1972	1996	2020	2043	2067	2090	2113	2136	2160
115	1961	1985	2010	2034	2058	2082	2106	2130	2154	2177	2201
120	1997	2022	2046	2071	2096	2120	2145	2169	2193	2217	2241
125	2032	2057	2082	2107	2132	2157	2182	2207	2231	2256	2280
130	2066	2092	2117	2143	2168	2194	2219	2244	2269	2294	2318
135	2099	2125	2152	2177	2203	2229	2255	2280	2305	2331	2356
140	2132	2159	2185	2211	2238	2264	2290	2316	2341	2367	2393
145	2165	2191	2218	2245	2271	2298	2324	2350	2377	2403	2429
150	2195	2223	2250	2277	2304	2331	2358	2385	2411	2437	2464
155	2226	2254	2282	2309	2337	2364	2391	2418	2445	2472	2498
160	2257	2285	2313	2341	2368	2396	2423	2451	2478	2505	2532
165	2286	2315	2343	2371	2399	2427	2455	2483	2511	2538	2566
170	2315	2344	2373	2402	2430	2458	2487	2515	2543	2571	2598
175	2344	2373	2402	2431	2460	2489	2518	2546	2574	2603	2631
180	2372	2402	2431	2461	2490	2519	2548	2577	2605	2634	2662
185	2400	2430	2460	2489	2510	2548	2578	2607	2636	2665	2693
190	2427	2458	2488	2518	2548	2577	2607	2637	2666	2695	2724
195	2454	2485	2512	2546	2576	2606	2636	2666	2695	2725	2754
200	2481	2515	2543	2573	2604	2634	2665	2695	2725	2754	2784
205	2507	2538	2570	2601	2631	2662	2693	2723	2753	2784	2814
210	2533	2565	2596	2627	2658	2689	2720	2751	2782	2812	2843
215	2558	2590	2622	2654	2685	2716	2748	2779	2810	2840	2871
220	2584	2616	2648	2680	2712	2743	2775	2806	2837	2868	2899
225	2608	2641	2673	2705	2738	2769	2801	2833	2864	2896	2927
230	2633	2666	2698	2731	2763	2795	2828	2860	2891	2923	2955
235	2657	2690	2723	2756	2789	2821	2854	2886	2918	2950	2982
240	2681	2714	2748	2781	2814	2846	2879	2912	2944	2976	3009
245	2704	2738	2772	2805	2838	2872	2905	2937	2970	3003	3035
250	2728	2762	2796	2829	2863	2896	2930	2963	2996	3029	3061
255	2751	2785	2819	2853	2887	2921	2954	2988	3021	3054	3087
260	2774	2808	2843	2877	2911	2945	2979	3012	3046	3079	3113
265	2796	2831	2866	2900	2935	2969	3003	3037	3071	3104	3138
270	2818	2854	2889	2923	2958	2993	3027	3061	3095	3129	3163
275	2841	2876	2911	2946	2981	3016	3051	3085	3120	3154	3188
280	2862	2898	2934	2969	3004	3039	3074	3109	3143	3178	3212
285	2884	2920	2956	2991	3027	3062	3097	3132	3167	3202	3237
290	2905	2942	2978	3014	3049	3085	3120	3156	3191	3226	3261

The Calories You Need (cont'd.)

69	70	71	72	73	74	75	76	77	78	79	80
2096	2118	2140	2162	2183	2205	2226	2248	2269	2291	2312	2333
2140	2162	2185	2207	2229	2251	2273	2295	2317	2339	2360	2382
2183	2205	2228	2251	2274	2296	2319	2341	2363	2385	2408	2430
2224	2247	2271	2294	2317	2340	2363	2386	2408	2431	2453	2476
2265	2288	2312	2336	2359	2383	2406	2429	2452	2475	2498	2521
2304	2329	2353	2377	2400	2424	2448	2472	2495	2519	2542	2565
2343	2368	2392	2417	2441	2465	2489	2513	2537	2561	2585	2608
2381	2406	2431	2456	2480	2505	2529	2554	2578	2602	2626	2651
2418	2443	2569	2494	2519	2544	2569	2594	2618	2643	2667	2692
2454	2480	2506	2531	2557	2582	2607	2633	2658	2683	2707	2732
2490	2516	2542	2568	2594	2620	2645	2671	2696	2721	2747	2772
2525	2551	2578	2604	2630	2656	2682	2708	2734	2760	2785	2811
2559	2586	2613	2639	2666	2692	2719	2745	2771	2797	2823	2849
2593	2620	2647	2674	2701	2728	2755	2781	2808	2834	2860	2886
2626	2654	2681	2708	2736	2763	2790	2817	2843	2870	2897	2923
2659	2686	2714	2742	2769	2797	2824	2852	2879	2906	2933	2960
2691	2719	2747	2775	2803	2831	2858	2886	2913	2941	2968	2995
2722	2751	2779	2807	2836	2864	2892	2920	2947	2975	3003	3030
2753	2782	2811	2839	2868	2896	2925	2955	2981	3009	3037	3065
2784	2813	2842	2871	2900	2929	2957	2986	3014	3043	3071	3099
2814	2843	2873	2902	2931	2960	2989	3018	3047	3075	3104	3132
2844	2873	2903	2933	2962	2991	3021	3050	3079	3108	3137	3165
2873	2903	2933	2963	2993	3022	3052	3081	3111	3140	3169	3198
2902	2932	2962	2993	3023	3053	3083	3112	3142	3171	3201	3230
2930	2961	2992	3022	3052	3083	3113	3143	3173	3203	3232	3262
2958	2989	3020	3051	3082	3112	3143	3173	3203	3233	3263	3293
2986	3017	3049	3080	3111	3141	3172	3203	3233	3264	3294	3324
3013	3045	3077	3108	3139	3170	3201	3232	3263	3294	3324	3355
3041	3072	3104	3136	3167	3199	3230	3261	3292	3323	3354	3385
3067	3099	3132	3163	3195	3227	3258	3290	3321	3352	3384	3415
3094	3126	3159	3191	3223	3255	3287	3318	3350	3381	3413	3444
3120	3153	3185	3218	3250	3282	3314	3346	3378	3410	3442	3473
3146	3179	3212	3244	3277	3309	3342	3374	3406	3438	3470	3502
3171	3205	3238	3271	3304	3336	3369	3401	3434	3466	3498	3530
3197	3230	3264	3297	3330	3363	3396	3429	3461	3494	3526	3559
3222	3255	3289	3323	3356	3389	3422	3455	3488	3521	3554	3586
3246	3280	3314	3348	3382	3415	3449	3482	3515	3548	3581	3614
3271	3305	3339	3373	3407	3441	3475	3508	3542	3575	3608	3641
3295	3330	3364	3398	3433	3467	3501	3534	3568	3602	3635	3668

week. This helps you identify where improvements can be made.

Here are the primary building blocks of HELP and the options available to you in each category. Rather than focus on what you may need to eliminate from your current menus, be willing to explore new foods and new ways to prepare them.

Block 1: Carbohydrates

Right under your nose, there is an intimate relationship going on between the carbohydrates in your body and your moods and emotions. This "love affair" is linked to your relationship with food—your eating habits, food cravings, and ability to lose weight. A fuller explanation of this love triangle and the role the hormone serotonin plays in it appears in Chapter 8. But here let's just say that complex carbohydrates are the mainstay of any weight loss program. Complex carbohydrates are found in whole-grain pasta, cereals, and breads; fruits and vegetables; and beans and legumes. Your body needs complex carbohydrates for energy production, and it craves them to relieve stress. (Fruits are the only carbohydrate foods that do not have stress-relieving qualities.) Most complex carbohydrates are also rich in fiber, which is essential for weight loss.

Simple carbohydrates—for example, white sugar and candy—provide lots of empty calories and burn quickly in the body. Those that don't burn turn into *fat*. Be aware that sugar is "hidden" in many products, especially processed foods. Read labels carefully. Sugar by any other name is just as sweet: sucrose, fructose, glucose, galactose, maltose, lactose, syrup, honey, cane sugar, and molasses are just a few of the ways sugar hides in your food. Many foods touted as "low fat" may have reduced their fat grams but are often packed with sugar as a way to retain the flavor lost by eliminating some of the fat. Sugar addiction is also a very significant problem for many people who want to lose weight. (See Chapter 4.)

Eating carbohydrates shuts off your appetite, but it doesn't happen immediately. When you feel a craving for carbohydrates, have your snack (e.g., fresh fruit, whole-grain crackers, or half a bagel), and then wait for about thirty minutes. That's how long it takes for the serotonin to have its calming, fulfilling effect. If your stomach is empty when you have the snack, it may take less time. If you continue to eat until you feel satisfied, you will probably eat many more calories than you need.

Block 2: Fiber

People used to snicker when they talked about fiber. This much-maligned part of food was "prescribed" for constipation and not much else. Today, however, we know that fiber is critical for successful weight loss. Increasing the amount of fiber in your diet adds bulk, which helps you feel full and puts the brakes on the urge to overeat. As fiber passes out of the body, it takes fat and toxins with it. Hemicellulose fiber, found in vegetables, fruits, and grains, is particularly helpful in weight loss.

The average American eats only 11 grams of fiber per day. To lose weight, you will need to increase the amount of dietary fiber, and perhaps add a fiber supplement, to reach the 20 to 35 grams recommended by most dietitians and physicians. Where your needs fall in that range depends on your current health and how much weight you want to lose. If you want to lose 30 pounds and you also have high cholesterol, for example, 35 grams per day is recommended. Fiber lowers cholesterol levels by binding to bile acids, the substances that make cholesterol in the liver.

How To Meet Your Fiber Needs

Increasing the fiber in your diet can be as easy as making a few substitutions. For example, white bread contains only 0.5 gram of fiber per slice; whole-grain breads can contain up to seven times as much. Whole fruit contains much more fiber than its juice alone. Red meat, chicken, fish, cheese, and milk contain no fiber. Hearty bean and legume dishes, pasta and marinara sauce, rice and vegetables—all can be substituted for meat and chicken and give you all the fiber and protein you need, without the fat and cholesterol! For example, consider the following sample menu.

HIGH-FIBER SUGGESTIONS
Breakfast
½ cup All-Bran cereal (10 g fiber; 70 calories; 0.5 g fat) with
½ cup nonfat rice or soy milk (0 g fiber; 45 calories; 0 g fat)
1 slice whole-grain bread (2 g fiber; 70 calories; 0.5 g fat) with
2 tsp. jam (0 g fiber; 38 calories; 0 g fat)
½ cup orange juice (0.5 g fiber; 55 calories; 0.2 g fat)

Lunch
Bean burrito with no-fat beans and whole-wheat tortilla (7 g fiber; 200 calories; 2.5 g fat)
½ cup Spanish rice (1 g fiber; 106 calories; 2.1 g fat)
½ cup canned mandarin oranges (4 g fiber; 46 calories; 0 fat)

Dinner
1 cup whole-wheat macaroni (5.4 g fiber; 210 calories; 2 g fat) with
½ cup "lite" marinara sauce (1 g fiber; 60 calories; 0 g fat)

½ cup butternut squash (4 g fiber; 40 calories; 0.1 g fat)
1 cup vegetarian vegetable soup (1 g fiber; 73 calories;
1 g fat)

Snacks

1 cup fresh blueberries (5 g fiber; 80 calories; 0.6 g fat)
2 cups air-popped popcorn (2 g fiber; 60 calories; 0.3 g
fat)

Your total: 42.9 g fiber; 1,173 calories; 9.8 g fat. See how
easy getting enough fiber can be? How does this sample plan
compare with the typical SAD diet?

SAD EATING
Breakfast

2 fried eggs (0 fiber; 208 calories; 15.6 g fat)
1 slice white bread (0 g fiber; 70 calories; 1.0 g fat) with
2 tsp. margarine (0 g fiber; 7.8 g fat; 66 calories)
1 sausage patty (0 g fiber; 100 calories; 8.4 g fat)

Lunch

3 oz. extra-lean hamburger (0 g fiber; 253 calories; 13.9 g
fat) with
1 slice American cheese (0 g fiber; 106 calories; 8.9 g fat)
on a hamburger roll (1 g fiber; 180 calories; 3 g fat)
10 french fries (2 g fiber; 158 calories; 8.3 g fat)

Dinner

½ fried chicken breast w/o skin (0 g fiber; 180 calories;
6.1 g fat)
½ cup mashed potatoes w/milk and marg. (1 g fiber; 130
calories; 6 g fat)
½ cup cole slaw w/mayo dressing (1 g fiber; 147 calories; 14.2 g fat)

Snacks

½ cup chocolate ice cream (1 g fiber; 150 calories; 8 g fat)

2 oz. light Pringles (0 g fiber; 300 calories; 16 g fat)

The total: only 6 g fiber, yet 117.2 g of fat and 2,048 calories! This SAD menu is also deficient in vitamins, minerals, and complex carbohydrates.

Use the following table to help you choose other high-fiber, low-calorie, low-fat foods for your HELP. Some of these foods are included in the sample HELP menus at the end of this chapter.

Fill'r Up with Fiber

Food	Portion	Calories	Fat (g)	Fiber (g)
Fiber One cereal	½ cup	64	1.1	10
Prunes, cooked	½ cup	113	0.2	10
Bran Chex	½ cup	136	1.2	9
Lentils, cooked	½ cup	116	0.8	8
Kidney beans, cooked	½ cup	112	0.5	8
Broccoli, fresh cooked	½ cup	22	0.3	2
Sweet potato, baked	1 small	118	0.1	7
Corn, whole kernel	½ cup	89	1.1	2
Macaroni, whole wheat	1 cup	220	2.0	5
Pear, fresh	1 med.	98	0.7	5
Chickpeas, canned	½ cup	135	2.1	5
Lima beans, cooked	½ cup	108	0.4	5
Beets, pickled	½ cup	75	0.1	4
Apple, w/peel	1 med	81	0.4	4
Squash, acorn, baked	½ cup	57	0.1	4
Peas, green, cooked	½ cup	67	0.2	4
Sauerkraut, canned	½ cup	22	0.2	4
Mango, fresh	1 med.	135	0.6	4
Orange, navel	1 med.	65	0.1	4

Pita, whole wheat	½ large	118	0.6	3.5
Artichoke, boiled	1 med.	53	0.2	3
Tangerine	1 med.	37	0.2	3
Strawberries, fresh	1 cup	45	0.6	3
Plum	1 med	36	0.4	3
Cantaloupe, fresh	1 cup	57	0.4	3
Spinach, cooked	½ cup	21	0.2	3
Cauliflower, cooked	1 cup	30	0.2	3
Rice, brown	½ cup	116	0.6	2
Asparagus, cooked	½ cup	22	0.3	2
Brussels sprouts	½ cup	30	0.4	2
Zucchini, cooked	½ cup	14	0.1	2
Eggplant, cooked	½ cup	13	0.1	2
Carrots, cooked	½ cup	35	0.1	2

Block 3: Fats

Americans love to eat fat, and considering that one-third of Americans are overweight, fat also loves Americans. If you are of average height and activity level, your daily calorie requirement is between 1,800 and 2,500 to meet your basic energy needs. Let's say you are also like the average American, who eats 85+ grams of fat per day. At 85 grams, that's 765 calories (9 calories/gram of fat × 85 grams = 765 calories). That doesn't leave many calories for protein and high-fiber carbohydrate foods. If, however, you eat 20 grams of fat per day, you get 180 calories from fat, or 10 percent of your total caloric needs. Now you are free to eat high-fiber vegetables, fruits, grains, and beans, which supply the fiber and nutrients your body needs to stay healthy and to lose weight. In fact, most people who switch from SAD to a HELP find they actually eat *more* food while consuming *fewer* calories.

All foods contain some fat—even celery—and all foods contain a combination of the three different types of fats: saturated, polyunsaturated, and monounsaturated. A fourth type—trans fatty acids—is manufactured. Each type of fat has a specific impact on the body.

- **Saturated fats** are most prevalent in meat, eggs, dairy products, and tropical oils. Compared with any other substances you consume, saturated fats cause the most significant increase in blood cholesterol.
- **Polyunsaturated fats,** found in vegetable oils, can lower blood levels of cholesterol a little, although polyunsaturated fats can raise triglyceride (fats in the blood) levels.
- **Monounsaturated fats** are found primarily in olives and olive oil and are considered to be safe if not heated.
- **Trans fatty acids** block cell respiration and cannot be processed effectively by the body. These villains are hidden in foods under the familiar words "hydrogenated" or "partially hydrogenated." This means they are manufactured chemically by adding hydrogen to vegetable oil to create a saturated (solid at room temperature) type of fat. Trans fatty acids are found in nearly all margarines and in many processed foods. In addition, heating these fats, as when foods are fried, makes then highly carcinogenic.

Now for the Good News

You need some fat in your diet for your bodily systems to function properly. The amount of healthy dietary fat right for you may be anywhere from 10 to 30 percent, depending on your health and the amount of weight you want to lose. On HELP, you *limit* all types of fat, not *eliminate* them, and you can begin to enjoy the weight loss benefits almost immediately. In addition, the majority of people who adopt a lower-fat eating plan also reverse the damage done to their blood vessels: blood cell clumping and vessel spasms stop, blood flow improves throughout the body, and platelet aggregation decreases.

To help you choose healthy fats, consider the following guidelines:

• Choose lower-fat foods like fruits, vegetables, whole grains, and legumes. Eliminate high-fat foods such as eggs, dairy products, candy, meat, fowl, fish, salad dressings, and fried foods. If you find it difficult to avoid dairy or meat products, limit yourself to low- or no-fat versions of dairy products. Treat meat, fowl, and fish as condiments—a few ounces a week, say, in a casserole, with stir-fry, or in pasta sauce.

• Read labels: avoid foods that contain hydrogenated oils or partially hydrogenated oils.

• Get the oil and fatty acids you need by eating small amounts of raw, whole foods such as avocados, seeds, and nuts, or take an essential fatty acid supplement such as evening primrose oil (see Chapter 6).

• Watch salt intake. Too much salt can make you crave fats.

• Beware of the lure of the no-fat and low-fat foods on the market. Read the labels carefully. No- or low-fat does not always mean significantly fewer calories. Many of these foods are loaded with sugar. While sugar has no fat, it has plenty of calories and can turn into fat if it is not burned off.

Block 4: Protein

Protein is constructed of amino acids, and the human body requires twenty-two amino acids to produce protein and other essential components. The body can manufacture thirteen of these amino acids; it must get the other nine from food. Though meat and dairy products are complete protein foods (they contain all nine essential amino acids), they also are high in fat and cholesterol and have no fiber. Most plant-based foods are not complete proteins, with the exception of soy protein, quinoa, and kamut (two grains). However, eating a variety of incomplete proteins during the day can fulfill your complete protein needs. For example: lentil soup with pasta; beans and brown rice; whole-wheat pasta with marinara and chickpeas; bean and tofu chili; bean burrito using a whole-wheat tortilla; oatmeal with low-fat soy milk or skim milk.

How much protein do you need? That depends on your body size. According to the National Research Council, you should figure on 0.45 grams of protein per pound of body weight; the World Health Organization (WHO) says about 3.5 grams. That translates into 56 grams for a 165-pound man or 48 grams for a 140-pound woman.

The fact is, while many Americans are worried about getting enough protein, most are consuming too much—more than 80 or 90 grams a day. Most of that excess protein is in the form of high-fat, high-cholesterol meat and dairy products. And too much protein intake is not healthy. Excess protein can cause kidney disorders as the kidneys must work overtime to handle the protein. Too much protein also promotes excretion of calcium (which leads to osteoporosis), causes gouty arthritis, and leads to fluid imbalance in the body.

Block 5: Nutrients

Most of the foods included in HELP are naturally high in many of the essential vitamins, minerals, enzymes, and other nutrients necessary for good health. It is beyond the scope of this book to list all the nutrients in the HELP foods. We recommend you consume organic fruits, vegetables, whole grains, and legumes when possible. Purchase foods that are free of artificial preservatives, colorings, and other additives. See Appendix B for books that include in-depth nutritional information on common foods.

Block 6: Water

You've probably heard it hundreds of times: you should drink six to eight 8-ounce glasses of water a day. If you are overweight, you need additional water—an extra 8-ounce glass of water for every 20 pounds of excess body weight—because overweight individuals have a greater metabolic rate.

Water is important for proper and efficient function of the kidneys and to help move fiber through the body. If the kidneys do not get enough water, the liver must take over. But the liver should be metabolizing stored fat into energy, and it can't do so if it's doing the kidneys' job.

While quantity of water is important, quality is critical. Use pure, bottled water when possible.

Foods You Can Live . . . and Lose With!

The HELP menu suggestions in this section have been gleaned from some of the most successful and effective weight loss and nutritional eating plans available today. Their results are supported by clinical studies and reflect the work of Drs. Gabriel Cousens, Martin Katahn, John McDougall, Dean Ornish, Nathan Pritikin, Michael Klaper, Melvyn Werbach, and others, such as Marilyn Diamond and Gary Null. These nutrition experts advocate an eating plan that is higher in carbohydrates (ranging from 50 to 80 percent) and lower in fat (10 to 30 percent), with protein recommendations in between (15 to 20 percent). They also strongly recommend the elimination of or drastic reduction in consumption of meat, fish, poultry, and dairy products to several ounces a week. To help you make the change, think Oriental! Treat these foods as condiments as the Japanese do, and soon you may find you don't need them at all.

Basically, these guidelines are suited for most people, not just those who want to lose weight, because they provide a comfortable range in which people can make adjustments to fit their unique needs. The meals are built around high-fiber foods that have no cholesterol, low fat, and lots of nutrients.

Tips for Transitioning to a Plant-Based Diet

If you are not already eating a plant-based diet, we want to help you make the transition easily and tastefully. That's why we've included some very flavorful and easy recipes in our menu section. If you're not ready to make a complete switch to plant-based eating, you can begin by reducing the amount of meat, poultry, and dairy products you include in your meals and the number of times per week that you have them. For example: a bit of slivered chicken in a vegetable stir-fry; a 2-ounce piece of fish with soba noodles or pasta marinara. A 3.5-ounce piece of chicken (breast, roasted) has 173 calories, 85 g of cholesterol, 0 g fiber, 30.9 g protein, 4.5 g fat; 3.5 oz. of lean ground beef has 272 calories, 24.7 g protein, 87 g cholesterol, 18.5 g fat, and 0 g fiber; and 3 oz. of baked mackerel has 223 calories, 20.3 g protein, 15.1 g fat, 64 g cholesterol, and 0 g fiber.

Be willing to experiment. Many tasty soy- and vegetable-based meat substitutes that look, taste, and have the texture of chicken, beef, and other items they are intended to replace are available in stores . . . and without the high fat and cholesterol.

Many people find it easier to make the switch if they eliminate poultry and meat but include fish occasionally. According to Andrew Weil, M.D., author of many natural health books, including *8 Weeks to Optimum Health,* oily, cold-water fish—salmon, kippers, mackerel, and sardines—are rich in omega-3 oils, which help reduce the risk of heart attack and improve blood fat levels. Most large ocean fish, shellfish, and freshwater fish are too contaminated to be safe for human consumption.

Not by White Bread Alone . . .

Insoluble fiber, found in the protective layer (bran) of grains, helps with weight loss. Modern milling processes remove this layer, but this is not so for whole grains. The following whole grains can be used in a variety of recipes (some included in this chapter). Most are rich in protein, B vitamins, vitamin E, thiamin, iron, magnesium, and zinc. They contain very little fat and no cholesterol.

AMARANTH: Used as a side dish, in salads, or popped like popcorn. Has a high protein content.

BARLEY: Used in soups, cold salads, pilafs, and as a hot cereal.

BUCKWHEAT: High in protein and contains all eight amino acids. Often used in pancakes and breads. It is not in the wheat family and so can be eaten by people allergic to or intolerant of wheat.

CORN: Most common types are sweet corn, popcorn, blue corn, polenta (finely ground cornmeal), hominy, grits, corn pastas, and masa harina (ground hominy to make tortillas and corn chips).

KAMUT: Used as a cereal or in grain salads.

MILLET: Excellent as cereal or in soups, stews, as a side dish, or in muffins.

OATS: Forms include oat groats, rolled oats, quick oats, and oat bran.

QUINOA: Most protein rich of all the grains; used in soups, stews, stuffing, and breads.

RICE: Varieties include brown, arborio, basmati, jasmine, Texamati, and wehani.

TRITICALE: Cross between rye and wheat and more nutritious than either grain alone. Used as cereal and in side dishes.

WHEAT: Forms include wheat berries (used as cereal or

like rice); bulgur (used to make taboule); couscous (used like rice). The gluten, which can be stripped from the wheat, is made into seitan, a high-protein meat substitute.

Healthy Substitutions

Instead Of . . .	Try This
Milk (for cereal or cooking)	Low-fat soy milk, rice milk, fruit juices
Cottage cheese (in recipes)	Crumbled tofu
Mayonnaise	Tofu mayonnaise (in stores)
Ice cream	Frozen fruit juice bars, Lite Tofutti, Light Mocha Mix
Eggs (for eating)	Tofu scrambled (recipe page 68)
Eggs (for cooking, baking)	Ener-G Egg Replacer; mashed banana, flaxseed, or applesauce
Meat, fish, and fowl	Whole grains, pasta, starchy vegetables, tofu and seitan (some recipes below)
Sodas	Plain or flavored mineral water, seltzer
Sweetened cereals	Any low-fat bran cereal with cinnamon or all-fruit jelly
Vegetable oils (in recipes)	Replace oil with water, mashed banana, or applesauce for moisture

Sample Menus
* = recipe included

Breakfast

#1: 1 ounce All-Bran (71 cal; 8.5 g fiber; 0.5 g fat)
     Served with ½ cup nonfat rice milk or soy milk (45 cal.; 0 g fat; 0 g fiber; 1 g protein)
     ½ cup blueberries (41 cal.; 0.3 fat; 1.0 fiber)

Optional: 1 slice whole-wheat toast (80 cal.; 2.4 g protein; 1.1 g fat; 1.6 g fiber) with 1 tbs. all-fruit jelly (32 cal.; 0 g protein, fat, fiber)
Herbal tea

#2:   Scrambled Squash and Tofu* (179 cal.)
Tempeh Strips* (170 cal.)
Optional: one slice whole-wheat bread with 1 tbs. all-fruit jelly (see Breakfast #1)
Herbal tea

#3:   French Toast* (2 slices) (191 cal.)
½ sliced banana (52 cal.; 0.6 g protein; 0.3 g fat; 0.3 g fiber)
Optional: 4 oz. orange juice (55 cal.; 1.7 protein; 0.1 fat; 0.13 fiber)

#4:   1 cup cream of wheat (134 cal.; 3.8 g protein; 0.5 g fat; 0 g fiber), served with ½ cup strawberries (22 cal; 0.4 g protein; 0.3 g fat; 0.4 g fiber)
1 slice whole-wheat bread with 1 tbs. all-fruit jelly (see Breakfast #1)
Herbal tea, coffee substitute

#5:   Brown Rice and Banana Pudding* (181 cal.)
1 cup cantaloupe (57 cal.; 1.4 g protein; 0.4 g fat; 0.50 g fiber)
Optional: add 1 banana (108 cal.; 1.2 g protein; 0.6 g fat; 0.57 g fiber)
Herbal tea, coffee substitute

Lunch
#1:   Hummus Sandwich* (195 cal.)
Served in whole-wheat pita (118 cal.; 2.4 g protein;

0.6 g fat; 3.5 g fiber) with tomato, onion, sprouts (negligible calories)
Optional: fresh fruit (select one or two): pear (98 cal.; 0.7 g fat; 2.3 g fiber); apple w/skin (80 cal.; 0.5 g fat; 4 g fiber); orange (64 cal.; 0.1 g fat; 4 g fiber); 1 cup fresh strawberries (45 cal.; 0.6 g fat; 3.4 g fiber)
Herbal tea, coffee substitute, iced tea with lemon

#2: 1 cup Greens and Potato Soup* (94 cal.)
$\frac{1}{2}$ cup black beans (112 cal.; 15.2 g protein; 0.2 g fat; 3.5 g fiber) mixed with 2 tbs. no-fat salsa (20 cal.; 0 g fat)
2 rice cakes (70 cal.; 0.4 g protein; 0.2 g fat; 0.40 g fiber)
6 oz. tomato juice (32 cal.; 1.4 g protein; 0.3 g fat; 0.72 g fiber)

#3: 1 large baked potato (104 cal.; 2.9 protein; 0.1 fat; 0.8 g fiber); stuffed with $\frac{1}{2}$ cup steamed broccoli (23 cal.; 2.3 g protein; 0.2 g fat; 2.3 g fiber) and 2 tbs. no-fat salsa (20 cal.; 0 g fat)
Optional: add Fava Bean Salad* (182 cal.)
Fresh fruit (see Lunch #1)
Herbal tea, coffee substitute, flavored seltzer water

#4: Roasted Eggplant* (69 cal.)
served in $\frac{1}{2}$ whole-wheat pita (118 cal.) with lettuce, tomato, onion if desired (negligible calories)
Rice Slaw* (102 cal.)
Herbal tea, coffee substitute, flavored seltzer water

#5: Carrot Soup* (123 cal.)
Low-fat vegetarian burger (depends on brand: cal. 90–110; 12–15 g protein; 0 g fat; 4 g fiber); served open-face on 1 slice whole-wheat bread (80 cal.)

Optional: use 2 slices of bread
Fresh fruit (see Lunch #1)
Herbal tea, coffee substitute, iced tea with lemon

Dinner

#1: Quick Szechwan Tofu* (166 cal.)
Served over ½ cup brown rice (109 cal.; 2.2 g protein;
0.8 g fat; 2 g fiber)
Optional: additional ½ cup rice
Baked papaya (88 cal.)
Herbal tea, coffee substitute, flavored seltzer water

#2: Harvest Chili* (212 cal.)
½ cup brown rice (109 cal.; 2.2 g protein; 0.8 g fat; 2
g fiber)
½ cup steamed green beans (22 cal.; 1.2 protein; 0.2
fat; 1.1 fiber)
Herbal tea, coffee substitute, flavored seltzer water

#3: 1 cup whole-wheat pasta (175 cal.; 7.5 protein; 0.8
fat; 5 g fiber); served with ½ cup no-fat marinara
sauce (50 cal.; 2 g protein; 0 g fat; 2 g fiber)
Salad with no-oil dressing, salsa, or lemon (include 1
cup romaine lettuce, ½ cup raw spinach, 1 small
tomato, 1 small carrot, shredded; ½ cup beets.
Approx. nutritional value: 84 cal.; 1.9 g protein; 0.7 g
fat; 2.7 g fiber)
Optional: add ¼ cup garbanzo beans to salad: 70
cal.; 3.5 g protein; 1.1 g fat; 2.5 g fiber)

#4: Vegetable Soup* (68 cal.)
Optional: 2 servings 10 oyster crackers (33 cal.; 1 g
fat; 0.7 g protein; 0 g fiber)
Collards and Tomatoes* (38 cal.)

Brown Rice and Banana Pudding* (181 cal.)
Herbal tea, coffee substitute, or 6 oz. tomato juice

#5:   Spicy Soba Noodles with Vegetables* (142 cal.)
1 cup Carrot Soup* (123 cal.)
½ cup steamed cauliflower (15 cal.; 1.2 g protein; 0.1
g fat; 1.0 g fiber)
Poached pears* (174 cal.)
Herbal tea, coffee substitute, or 6 oz. tomato juice

Snacks
Bean/Garlic Dip* w/raw vegetables
Air-popped popcorn (per cup: 31 cal.; 1 g protein; 0.3 g
fat; 0.30 g fiber)
Fresh fruit

Recipes for Health

See Appendix B, Sources and Suggested Readings, for a comprehensive list of books containing healthy recipes.

Tempeh Strips
Makes 12–16 strips

*Spray oil
8 oz. tempeh, sliced thin
¼ cup brown rice syrup
2 tbs. soy sauce*

Preheat oven to 450°F. Lightly spray oil on a baking sheet and place strips on sheet. Drizzle with syrup and soy sauce. Season with pepper and lightly spray the sheet again. Bake 5–10 minutes, until lightly browned. Turn strips over and bake for another 5 minutes.

Per serving (3 strips): 170 cal.; 10 g protein; 4 g fat; 3 g fiber

French Toast

   1 banana, peeled
   4 strawberries (or 1/3 cup blueberries)
   1/3 cup apple juice
   1/2 tsp. cinnamon
   4 slices whole-wheat or 7-grain bread

Place first four ingredients in a blender and process until smooth. Soak the bread in the mixture and cook on both sides on a nonstick griddle or one sprayed with oil.

Per serving (2 slices): 191 cal.; 6 g protein; 2 g fat; 5 g fiber

Rice Slaw
Makes 8 cups

   2 cups brown rice, cooked
   1/2 small red cabbage, shredded
   2 carrots, julienned
   1 small red onion, sliced thin
   1 medium fennel, sliced thin
   1 tsp. each caraway seed and pepper
   1/4 cup each balsamic vinegar and olive oil
   2 tbs. each Dijon mustard and olive oil

Tip: Reduce calories and fat by eliminating all but 3 tbs. of olive oil.

Combine all ingredients and mix well. Let stand for 30 minutes before serving.

Per one-cup serving: 102 cal.; 2 g protein; 4 g fat; 2 g fiber

Vegetable Soup
Serves 4

   1 small eggplant
   3 medium onions, chopped

2 cloves garlic, chopped
4 cups water
2 small zucchini, chopped
3 tomatoes, chopped
1 tbs. curry powder
1/2 tsp. turmeric

Preheat oven to 400°F. Pierce the eggplant in several places and put it on an ungreased baking sheet. Bake 15–20 minutes until soft. Remove from oven; peel and chop when cooled. In the meantime, cook onion and garlic in 1/2 cup water until soft, about 5 minutes. Stir in eggplant and all remaining ingredients. Bring to a boil; reduce heat to simmer for 15 minutes.

Per serving: 68 cal.; 3 g protein; 1 g fat; 4.3 g fiber

Greens and Potato Soup
Makes 8 cups

1 tbs. canola oil
2 cloves garlic, minced
4 leeks, sliced, soaked, and drained
4 medium potatoes, peeled and diced
4 cups vegetable broth
2 cups chopped spinach or mustard greens
Salt and pepper to taste

Sauté garlic and leeks in oil for 5 minutes. Add potatoes and broth; simmer for 25 minutes. Add greens and simmer for 10 minutes. Purée the mixture in a food processor or blender. Season to taste.

Per cup: 94 cal.; 1.1 g protein; 1.7 g fat; 3.4 g fiber

Carrot Soup
Makes 4 one-cup servings

1 tbs. olive oil

1 medium onion, sliced
½ tsp. each salt, coriander, tarragon, and marjoram
3 cups peeled and sliced carrots (about 6 carrots)
2½ cups vegetable broth
2 tbs. orange juice
1 large sweet potato, peeled and sliced (about 1½ cups)

Heat oil in saucepan and sauté onion and salt for about 5 minutes. (*Tip:* Save calories and fat by steaming onion and salt in a little bit of water.) Add other spices and cook 5 minutes. Stir in carrots, potato, and broth. Bring to a boil, reduce heat and simmer, covered, for 20 minutes. Add orange juice and pour soup into a blender and purée.

Per one-cup serving, using oil: 123 cal.; 5 g protein; 2.5 g fat; 4.2 g fiber

Spicy Soba Noodles with Vegetables
Makes 4 one-cup servings

8 oz. soba noodles
2 tbs. each olive oil, minced garlic, tamari, water
3 medium carrots, sliced thin
1 tbs. fresh ginger, minced
2 bunches fresh spinach, stemmed and chopped coarsely
¼ tsp. ground cloves
1 tsp. grated orange

Cook noodles until slightly firm. Drain, rinse with cold water, and set aside. In a skillet, sauté garlic for 3 minutes. Add carrots, ginger, and cloves and cook for 5 minutes. Add spinach, tamari, and water. Cook until spinach is wilted, about 2–3 minutes. Add noodles, mix, and cook until heated.

Per serving (1 cup): 142 cal.; 5 g protein; 3.6 g fat; 5.2 g fiber

Roasted Eggplant

Makes about 24 slices, or 6 servings

2 large eggplant, cut into thin slices
2 tbs. each olive oil and balsamic or red wine vinegar
Salt and pepper to taste

Preheat oven to 450°F. In a large bowl, mix the slices with the oil until coated. Lay slices on a baking sheet and roast in the oven for 15 minutes. Sprinkle with vinegar, salt, and pepper. Use for sandwiches, stuffed in pita, or as a side dish.

Per serving (4 slices): 69 cal.; 1 g protein; 2.1 g fat; 3.7 g fiber

Quick Szechwan Tofu

Makes 4 servings

6 cloves garlic, minced
1 tbs. oil
1 tbs. fresh gingerroot, minced
2 tbs. each tomato paste, cornstarch
14 oz. firm tofu, cubed
2 carrots, diced
2 zucchini, diced
¼ cup soy sauce
1 cup vegetable broth
1 yellow onion, diced
15-oz. can straw mushrooms, or 1 lb. sliced fresh
   mushrooms
½ cup rice vinegar

In a wok or large skillet, sauté garlic and ginger in oil for 1 minute on high heat. Add tofu and stir occasionally for 5 minutes. Add zucchini, carrots, and onion and lower heat. In a bowl, combine soy, broth, vinegar, tomato paste, and cornstarch and add to wok. Raise heat and simmer until sauce thickens, about 3 minutes. Add mushrooms before serving.

Per serving: 166 cal.; 11 g protein; 7 g fat; 2 g fiber

Harvest Chili
Makes 10 servings

2 onions, chopped
4 carrots, chopped
4 stalks celery, chopped
4 cloves garlic, minced
6 cups water
2 tbs. fresh oregano or 2 tsp. dried
1/2 tsp. each salt and black pepper
1/2 cup each dry couscous and dry bulgur
2 jalapeños, seeded and diced
2 zucchini, sliced
1 cup each corn kernels, green beans
8 tomatoes, diced
3 cups cooked black or pinto beans, or use both

In a large pot, cook onion, carrots, celery, and garlic in 1 cup water for 15 minutes. Add remaining ingredients and bring to a boil. Reduce heat and simmer 1 hour.

Per serving: 212 cal; 10 g protein; 1 g fat; 10.7 g fiber

Collards and Tomatoes
Serves 4

1 tsp. olive oil
1 lb. collards or kale, chopped
2 ripe tomatoes, chopped
2 tsp. lemon juice
1/2 tsp. garlic powder
1/4 tsp. mustard powder

Sauté all the ingredients together 3–5 minutes.
Per serving: 38 cal.; 2 g protein; 2 g fat; 3 g fiber

Fava Bean Salad
Serves 3

1 small onion and one stalk celery, chopped
1 tbs. olive oil
19-oz. can fava beans, drained
1 ripe tomato, chopped
1 tsp. each: lemon juice and cumin
1/8 tsp. black pepper

Sauté onion in oil. Add remaining ingredients and cook for 10 minutes. Serve cold as a salad or hot over rice, pasta, or other grain.
Per serving: 182 cal.; 10 g protein; 5 g fat; 3 g fiber

Scrambled Squash and Tofu
Serves 2

1 tbs. olive oil
1 medium zucchini or yellow squash
1 small onion, minced
1/4 tsp. pepper
2 tbs. no-fat salsa
1/2 lb. tofu, crumbled
1/4 tsp. soy sauce

Sauté the zucchini, onion, and pepper in oil until the squash is soft. Add the tofu, soy sauce, and salsa and saute 3–5 minutes.
Per serving: 179 cal.; 11 g protein; 13 g fat; 3 g fiber.
Tip: Reduce calories and fat by steaming the vegetables in water.

Hummus

Makes 2 cups, or four ½-cup servings

2 cups cooked garbanzo beans
⅛ cup tahini
1 tbs. olive oil
2 cloves garlic, minced
1 tbs. lemon juice
½ tsp. each: cumin, coriander seed
Salt to taste

Combine all ingredients in food processor or blender and process until smooth.

Per ½-cup serving: 195 cal.; 7.5 g protein; 6.3 g fat; 5.4 g fiber

Brown Rice and Banana Pudding

Makes 4 one-cup servings

1 cup brown rice
3 cups no-fat rice milk
3 bananas, mashed
1 tsp. vanilla extract
½ tsp. nutmeg

Combine all ingredients in a casserole, cover, and bake at 350°F for 75 minutes.

Per serving: 181 cal.; 7 g protein; 1 g fat; 2 g fiber

Baked Papaya

Makes 4 servings

2 ripe papayas
4 tbs. frozen orange juice concentrate
½ tsp. cinnamon

Preheat oven to 350°F. Skin the papayas, slice, and lay pieces in a baking dish. Sprinkle papaya with juice concentrate and cinnamon. Bake for 20 minutes. Serve hot.

Per serving (½ papaya): 88 cal.; 1 g protein; 0.5 g fat; 1 g fiber

Poached Pears
Makes 4 servings

2½ cups apple juice
Juice and zest of 1 lemon
4 firm Bosc pears
1 tbs. fennel seeds

Mix juice and lemon in saucepan. Peel and core pears and put pears and peelings in the pan. Bring to a boil, reduce heat, and let pears cook 3–5 minutes. Remove pears and chill. Strain liquid and return to pot with fennel and lemon zest. Cook on medium heat for 10 minutes or until thickened. Pears can be heated in sauce or served cold with warm sauce.

Per serving: 174 cal.; 1 g protein; 0 g fat; 5 g fiber

Bean/Garlic Dip
Serves 2

⅓ lb. green beans
2 cloves garlic, minced
½ tsp. onion powder
1 tsp. soy sauce
1½ tbs. tahini

Steam beans for 10 minutes in about 1 cup of water until tender. Rinse beans in cold water. Place remaining ingredients in a blender. Add cooked beans. Blend until smooth.

Per serving: 69 cal.; 3 g protein; 4 g fat; 3 g fiber

Tips for Eating Out

So many Americans eat out that we need to address the challenges of restaurant food. Many restaurants advertise that they serve healthy, "heart healthy," and vegetarian foods. Ethnic restaurants such as Chinese, Japanese, Thai, and Indian are usually good choices for such meals. Regardless of the type of restaurant you go to, however, don't be afraid to ask questions of the wait staff and cooks if necessary. Not everyone defines "healthy" in the same way. Don't hesitate to request specific items. You don't need to give a long explanation; you can simply say, "I'm on a special diet." Ask that your vegetables be steamed or roasted with herbs and without oil. Ask what is in their soup stock (many hide oils and animal fat). Do they have whole-grain breads and pastas and brown rice? Do they use MSG or lard? Bring your own salad dressing from home when you go out to eat, or ask for lemon, vinegar, and herbs on the side. Salsa is an excellent condiment to use instead of gravies or oils on vegetables, baked potatoes, pasta, and grains. Ask for a small bowl on the side.

You may want to call ahead before you waste your time driving to a restaurant that has little to offer you. Call during off hours; no one will have the time to answer your questions adequately if you call during lunch or dinner.

American Cancer Society Guidelines On Diet, Nutrition, and Cancer

- Maintain a healthy body weight for your height and structure
- Eat a varied diet each day that includes an assortment of fruits and vegetables and other high-fiber foods such as whole-grain cereals and legumes
- Reduce total fat intake to 30 percent or less

- Limit or eliminate consumption of alcoholic beverages
- Limit or eliminate consumption of foods that are smoked or preserved with salt or nitrites

A switch to healthy eating habits is a lifetime commitment, so you'll want to make it easy, fun, and tasty. As you make the transition, you'll be adding new foods as well as learning how to prepare old favorites in new ways. There are dozens of books and thousands of recipes for tasty, nutritious, high-fiber, lower-fat foods that are easy to make (see Appendix B).

A positive attitude is important when making the transition to new eating habits. Banish any thoughts that you are depriving yourself and focus on the new discoveries and the great way you will feel and look as you not only lose pounds but gain self-confidence, energy, and better health.

CHAPTER FOUR

Beating Your Craving
for Sugar

Many people have a "sweet tooth," a craving for cookies, candy, ice cream, cake, pie . . . anything sweet. But often it is much more than just a desire: it is an addiction. In fact, along with alcohol and tobacco, sugar is one of the most addicting substances known. Some nutritionists go so far as to claim that sugar is the most common form of dependence in our society. Regardless of who is correct, sugar causes serious cravings in many people and is a significant problem for people who want to lose weight.

What Is Sugar?

Sugar is a carbohydrate, which means it is composed of carbon, hydrogen, and oxygen. Starches also are carbohydrates, yet there are some very significant differences in the way sugar and starches affect human metabolism. Without getting into the intricacies of how sugar and starches are formed and metabolized, let's just say that there are simple sugars (or simple carbohydrates), of which sucrose, or white sugar, is the most common. When many simple sugars combine, they form starches, or complex carbohydrates. (See Chapter 3.)

Because of its simple nature, sugar is metabolized very rapidly by the body. That's why many people will reach for a candy bar or cookies when they want a quick pick-me-up. But shortly thereafter comes the letdown, as if someone has "pulled the plug" and drained them of their energy. Complex carbohydrates, however, metabolize more slowly and provide a more even flow of energy.

How Much Sugar We Eat and Why

The average American consumes thirty to forty teaspoons of sugar a day. Impossible, you say; you use only a teaspoon in your coffee, another in your cereal, and there's probably several in those cookies you like so much, but how does that add up to thirty or more?

To understand how it all adds up, you should know a bit about the human hankering for sugar. A liking for sweet things is something humans share with many creatures in the animal kingdom. For millennia, the desire was satisfied with fruit and honey. Yet people's liking for sweets has evolved as technology and food processing have progressed, and the evolution has to do with acquired tastes.

There are four basic tastes—bitter, sweet, salty, and sour—and our taste buds can recognize only these four. When you place food into your mouth, the taste buds send signals to the brain, which then distinguishes among the various shades of tastes, leaving you with a distinct taste for that food item.

The first taste a human infant is able to detect is sweet, which can be recognized almost at birth. (A taste for salt doesn't develop until about age 4 months.) Conditioning for sweetness begins almost immediately for many infants. Though mothers' milk is not sweet, many mothers resort to formulas and then to commercially available baby foods, which contain sugars and added carbohydrates. According to medical researcher Dr. John Yudkin, author of *Pure White and Deadly,* "If . . . people are laying the foundations for serious disease in later life by encouraging the development of a sweet tooth in children, this may be doing them even more harm than if they were encouraged to begin smoking at the age of twelve or fifteen."

Nowadays there is added sugar in some form in nearly every processed food on the shelves: from ketchup to breakfast cereals (even the unsweetened ones); from soup to canned vegetables; and from frozen waffles to spaghetti sauce. It is estimated that Americans consume about 125 grams of sucrose daily and about 70 grams of fructose, or fruit sugar, per day. This represents a tremendous change in our eating habits: the "best guess" of experts is that primitive peoples ate 5 grams of natural sugars per day. Since the mid-1800s, our consumption of sugar has increased more than fiftyfold. This excessive amount of sugar is being linked with the rise in obesity, diabetes, and other diseases. And the desire for sugar remains strong: in fact, manufacturers add sugar because it enhances the flavor of the food and because it leaves you wanting more: it is addictive.

The Addiction Process

An addiction—the physical, psychological (or both) dependence on a substance or behavior—can occur when something you do stimulates your adrenaline flow and makes you feel good. To make the good feeling return, you ingest the substance or repeat the behavior again and again. Over time, your mind-body depends on that adrenaline "kick." You may get the kick from running, smoking a cigarette, drinking coffee, or eating something sweet. With a sugar addiction, the process may occur subtly because you may not realize how much sugar you are really consuming in processed foods.

When you ingest sucrose, your blood sugar level rises quickly. To bring the sugar level down, insulin pours into your bloodstream. However, the body may release more insulin than it needs, which ultimately causes the adrenal glands to send out adrenaline. If you continue to eat a lot of sugar, your body will keep pumping out adrenaline. The result: you like the feeling, even though you probably are not conscious of it, and eventually you may become addicted to sugar.

Some experts believe that if we constantly stimulate the sweetness taste buds, we may produce more of them, which in turn will increase the cravings for sweets. They even suggest that the culinary customs of Oriental and other cultures to combine sweet and sour helps prevent a craving for sugar.

Breaking Away from Sugar

How do you know if you have a sugar addiction? Examine your eating and drinking habits.

- On a daily basis, do you eat or drink foods or beverages that contain sugar?
- Do you experience an intense, even uncontrollable craving for these foods?
- Do you experience feelings of nervousness or anxiety, or do you get headaches or other physical symptoms if you do not consume these foods daily?
- Do you find yourself thinking about these foods and worrying about not being able to get them (e.g., you're on a trip or in a meeting and cannot get to your ''stash'' of candy)?

A "yes" response to the first question is common; but if it is combined with a "yes" from one or more of the next three, you are addicted to sugar. One of the most significant signs that sugar is addicting is the withdrawal many people experience once they eliminate sugar from their diet. Going "cold turkey" often results in headache, shakiness, fainting, abdominal cramps, palpitations, and even vomiting. People become nervous, jittery, and mentally confused and unable to concentrate. These are the same symptoms associated with withdrawal from alcohol and other drugs.

It's important that you know these symptoms are only temporary and vary in intensity depending on your level of addiction.

Breaking Sugar Addiction Naturally

An addiction to sugar can make it impossible for you to lose weight until it is resolved. For that reason, some medical practitioners prescribe a sugar withdrawal program which involves taking specific supplements that help eliminate cravings for sugar. An example of such a program is discussed on page 78. Many physicians use a similar withdrawal program, with some adding biotin (3,000 mg a day) or increasing chromium intake to 1,000 mg per day. Your physician can determine the appropriate balance of substances for your needs.

Elimination of sugar cravings often is the catalyst for a successful weight loss and maintenance program. Withdrawal from sugar automatically reduces caloric intake and, if you have a yeast infection, is critical to successfully eradicating that condition as well. Ridding the body of sugar's toxicity leads to increased energy, which promotes exercise. It also allows you to more easily identify any food allergies or intolerances you may be experiencing, as a sugar dependency can mask these food-related problems.

Sugar cravings have also been linked with serotonin

levels: a low level of this hormone is associated with increased cravings. Foods that help raise serotonin levels include starchy complex carbohydrates such as potatoes and whole-grain cereals and pastas, and foods that slowly release their energy into the bloodstream, such as apples and popcorn. Substituting these foods for high-sugar, high-calorie candy, cookies, and soda can help you kick the sugar habit.

Sugar Withdrawal Program

VITAMIN C: (take in crystalline or powder form as sodium ascorbate or calcium ascorbate). Vitamin C is the foundation of a sugar detoxification protocol. It helps eliminate and modify withdrawal symptoms and provides adrenal support.

→**Dose:** 4,000 mg/tsp.; 1 tsp. every 2 to 4 hours during the detoxification period. Detoxification lasts from three to seven days. Continue this regimen until sugar cravings disappear. Then reduce vitamin C intake to twice daily.

GLUTAMINE: An amino acid that reduces cravings for sugar, drugs, and alcohol. It also helps repair intestinal tissue and enhances its function.

→**Dose:** 500 mg four times a day between meals

CHROMIUM: Also known as Glucose Tolerance Factor, or GTF, helps the body burn fat and lower serum lipid levels. It also helps insulin remove sugar from the blood more efficiently.

→**Dose:** 200 mcg twice a day

Source: With permission of Hunter Yost, M.D.

Benefits of Breaking the Habit

The most immediate advantages of breaking the sugar habit are usually weight loss and an increase in energy. As you eliminate those excessive, empty calories from your menu, you will replace them with fulfilling, nutritious foods. You will not go hungry: quite the contrary. Sugary foods leave you feeling unfulfilled; high-fiber, complex carbohydrates satisfy hunger, plus provide your body with the raw materials to keep your energy level on a more even keel. No more sugar highs and lows!

Researchers have found that a high consumption of sugar is associated with a lower resistance to infections, such as the common cold and flu. People who experience a rapid rise in blood sugar levels after they eat foods high in sucrose, fructose, or other simple sugars have less ability to fight infections. This reduced ability to resist bacteria lasts for about four to five hours after eating the sugary food. If you eat sweet foods or drink sugary beverages routinely throughout the day, your ability to ward off infection may be compromised all the time.

Elimination of a sugar addiction can be a tremendous boost to your effort to lose weight, as well as a move toward better health and well-being. Become a label reader: know your food and what you're really bringing home to your table. Buy whole, organic foods when possible. When you break away from the sugar habit, you will lose weight and get off the roller coaster of high and low energy.

CHAPTER FIVE

Chromium Picolinate and Other Thermogenic Agents

If someone offered you a product that could boost the rate at which your body burned fat without your losing muscle tone, chances are good you would at least want to know more about it, if not be among the first in line to try it. The fact is that several substances currently on the market, including chromium picolinate, caffeine, and ephedrine (mahuang), are being used for these very purposes. Collectively these items are called *thermogenic* agents. The process known as **thermogenesis,** which means "creation of heat," is the method by which the body transforms the food you eat into heat. In some people, food intake may stimulate up to a 40 percent increase in the production of heat; these individuals tend to be thin. In others, heat production may be 10 percent or less, and the extra food energy is stored instead of burned or metabolized. (Thermogenesis is actually a part of the complex metabolic process; but for the sake of simplicity, we use the terms *thermogenesis* and *metabolic rate* interchangeably.)

Everyone has his or her own thermogenic, or metabolic, rate, which is genetically determined. That does not mean, however, that you cannot change the rate at which fat is burned. Exercise is one way you can increase metabolism; the use of natural thermogenic substances is another. In this chapter we discuss the most popular and reportedly the most effective of these natural substances, including how to use them and controversies surrounding their use. First, however, let's look at the process these thermogenic agents are meant to change.

Metabolic Rate

The number of calories your body needs while at rest, before allowing for physical activity, is known as the basal (base) metabolic rate, or BMR. (The calorie count you calculated in Chapter 3 gives you an estimate of your BMR plus calories needed to maintain your current weight.) When you first reduce your caloric intake, your body loses protein and glycogen—both of which contain water—and salt. This is what occurs when people talk about "losing water weight." As your body adjusts to fewer calories and tries to reserve energy, the amount of energy your body needs to function decreases, and your body produces more fat-storing enzymes as a "survival" tactic. The fewer calories you consume, the lower your metabolic rate will go.

Your body now has less ability to metabolize fat because it is losing muscle, and muscle requires more calories than does fat. You also now have a larger supply of very efficient fat-storing enzymes. The 2,000 calories that once allowed you to maintain your weight now add pounds. Researchers at Rockefeller University in New York report that this change in metabolism happens to everyone when they lose weight. In a March 1995 study published in the *New England Journal of Medicine* by the Rockefeller team, it was shown that when dieting research volunteers lost about 10 percent of their weight, the overall calories burned decreased an average of 15 percent. If you go on a more severe diet, your metabolic rate can decrease by as much as 40 percent. These findings support the recommendation to set individual goals to lose 10 percent of your body weight (see Chapter 3, under A Few Words on Calories). The conclusion is that the body alters its metabolic rate to gravitate toward a natural weight, or set point.

Thermogenesis: Burn, Baby, Burn

Researchers have discovered that certain natural substances may trigger your body's thermostat and cause it to burn more fat. These substances can be used to supplement your eating and exercise program to boost your weight loss efforts. Some of these agents include chromium picolinate, ephedra (mahuang), cayenne, Co-Q-10, gammalinolenic acid, *Gymnema sylvestre* extract, and other substances commonly added to chromium or ephedra formulations, such as hydroxycitric acid, kola nuts, green tea, and guarana extract. Now let's explore these supplements.

Chromium Picolinate

Chromium is an essential mineral found naturally in the body and in some foods, such as Brewer's yeast, whole wheat, rye, broccoli, mushrooms, potatoes, green peppers, and apples. It is an essential part of the *Glucose Tolerance Factor* (GTF), a molecule that is critical in enhancing insulin function and the use of glucose by the body. Thus, chromium's primary roles as part of GTF are to facilitate proper carbohydrate metabolism and to help insulin as it makes blood sugar available to the cells.

Your body releases insulin when you digest carbohydrates. At the same time, it also releases chromium as a helper, or *cofactor,* to insulin. Insulin is responsible for keeping body fat low and lean muscle high. Chromium increases the absorbability of insulin, thereby assisting in the reduction of body fat and the promotion of lean muscle.

Proponents of chromium picolinate supplementation (the most popular form of this supplement mineral) claim it can help people lose weight by boosting their metabolic rate. This claim is based on a study performed by Gary Evans, a chemist at Bemidji State University in Minnesota. The study involved forty-one athletes, some of whom took 200 mcg of chromium (the standard supplemental dose) and some who took a placebo. Those who took chromium had increased muscle mass and a reduction in percentage of body fat. Based on these results, Evans patented chromium picolinate as a dietary supplement in the late 1980s. Subsequent studies have supported this finding.

How Much to Take

Although no Recommended Daily Allowance (RDA) has been established for chromium, experts with the National Academy of Sciences believe 50 to 200 mcg per day is adequate, while others recommend 200 to 400 mcg for women and 400 to 600 mcg for men. It is estimated that between 25 and 50 percent of Americans are deficient in chromium. This is primarily due to poor chromium supplies in the soil and the amount of refined foods Americans consume, because processing strips food of essential nutrients, including chromium. People who eat the Standard American Diet (SAD)—high-fat, high-sugar, with many refined flour and sugar products—often are not only overweight but are also deficient in chromium.

Forms of Chromium Supplements

Chromium supplements are available in several forms—chromium yeast, chromium oxide and trioxide, chromium gluconate, GTF or pure niacin-bound chromium, chromium chelate, and chromium picolinate. The latter two forms are better absorbed than the others.

Consumers Beware

Not all studies of chromium picolinate have shown the supplement to be beneficial. One such study was conducted by Hank Lukaski, research leader at the U.S. Department of Agriculture Human Nutrition Research Center in Grand Forks, North Dakota. He reported on April 29, 1994, that "Chromium picolinate has no effect on building muscle, reducing body fat, changing body composition, decreasing weight or increasing strength."

A *Consumer Reports* article in November 1995 stated that much of the research conducted on chromium picolinate has been done by the patent holder, while most studies conducted by independent researchers have failed to support the weight loss claims. The FDA has expressed concern over reports of adverse effects, including irregular heartbeat, and animal studies suggest that taking too much chromium picolinate can be harmful.

A few study results indicate that dosages of 1,000 mcg or greater over weeks or months may be toxic and cause iron deficiencies or disrupt insulin's activity. Researchers generally agree that once the body gets the chromium it needs, the excess is eliminated in the urine and feces, which means you could be flushing money down the toilet.

Ephedra

The controversial herbal remedy ephedra *(Ephedra sinica),* also known as mahuang (Chinese ephedra), Mormon tea (the American species), and epitonin, is a branching shrub often used as a dietary aid. Its active ingredients—ephedrine, pseudoephedrine, and norpseudoephedrine—are central nervous system stimulants that are less potent than amphetamines. Ephedrine's role in weight loss is to stimulate the beta receptors on the fat cells, which in turn activates thermogenesis, burns stored fat, and generates energy, according to researchers in the *International Journal of Obesity*. Indeed, several studies indicate that ephedrine, when taken alone or used along with other thermogenic substances such as caffeine, kola nuts (which contain caffeine), and salicylates (aspirin), promotes greater weight loss than placebo (see Combinations of Ephedrine and Other Substances, page 86). Chinese ephedra contains significant amounts of ephedrine and is preferred over the other species for weight loss. The American species, Mormon tea, is richer in norpseudoephedrine. Mormon tea is so named because the Mormons used it as a coffee and tea substitute when they were first introduced to the herb in 1847.

Dosing
The usual dose of ephedra for weight loss is as follows (information on how to make herbal preparations appears in Chapter 6). To prepare a decoction, add 1 ounce of dried mahuang to eight ounces of boiling water. Reduce heat and let simmer for 15 minutes. Drink up to 2 cups per day. To use a tincture, add ¼ to 1 teaspoon to water and drink up to three times a day. If you purchase a commercial preparation, follow the package directions.

Consumers Beware
The use of ephedra raises several health safety issues; thus it should be taken only under a doctor's care. Conventional medical investigators claim that pseudoephedrine, a chemical currently used in commercial cold formulas, is safer than ephedrine. Ephedrine stimulates the heart, raises blood pressure, increases metabolic rate and perspiration and urine production, and reduces the secretion of saliva and stomach acids. It also can cause paranoid psychoses, coronary spasm,

convulsions, respiratory depression, and coma. Anyone with a heart condition or any neurologic disorder should avoid using this herb. Herbalists note that use of the entire ephedra plant is safer than either ephedrine or pseudoephedrine. British herbalist Michael McIntyre, author of *Herbal Medicine for Everyone,* explains that while pure ephedrine "markedly raises blood pressure . . . the whole plant actually reduces blood pressure."

A common practice is to combine ephedrine with other substances to boost the herb's effects. Combinations of ephedrine, phenylpropanolamine (PPA; an ephedrine alkaloid found in weight control products and over-the-counter cold and allergy formulas; see Chapter 2), and caffeine are common. We look at some of these combinations below.

Consumers may have the ephedra issue decided for them. In June 1997, the U.S. government announced that it would dramatically reduce the amount of ephedra that could be put into any dietary supplement and ban the marketing of any weight loss or bodybuilding products that contained ephedrine. This decision was made after at least 17 people died and more than 800 became ill after taking weight loss products containing ephedrine.

People with heart disease, diabetes, glaucoma, high blood pressure, hyperthyroidism, women who are pregnant or nursing, and anyone who is taking medications that raise blood pressure or that cause anxiety or insomnia should not use ephedra.

Combinations of Ephedrine and Other Substances

The weight loss action of ephedrine can be greatly enhanced when it is combined with caffeine-containing herbs like kola nut, guarana extract, and green tea. Studies published in the *International Journal of Obesity* and other journals note that a combination of ephedrine, caffeine, and theophylline (a substance similar to caffeine and found in tea leaves) is more than twice as effective as ephedrine alone for increasing the metabolic rate in overweight individuals. The dosages that led to this response were 22 mg of ephedrine and 80 mg of caffeine per day (the approximate amount of caffeine in one cup of coffee), which are the levels recommended by Michael T. Murray, N.D., author of *Natural Alternatives to Over-the-Counter and Prescription Drugs* and *Natural Alternatives for Weight Loss.* By comparison, 800 mg of guarana extract, taken from a plant that is found primarily in the Amazon jungle, is equivalent to 32 mg of caffeine.

Dr. Murray recommends taking ephedrine-caffeine combinations early in the day and avoiding any other products that contain caffeine while taking any thermogenic agent. If you have high blood pressure or heart disease or are taking antidepressants, consult with your doctor before starting any thermogenic therapy that contains ephedrine. Possible side effects from an ephedrine-caffeine combination include dizziness, anxiety, insomnia, high blood pressure, and tremors.

An herbal form of aspirin, willow bark extract, is sometimes added to an ephedrine–herbal caffeine combination. Such a remedy is about twice as effective as ephedrine alone at increasing the metabolic rate. Beware of any combinations containing ephedrine, PPA, and caffeine, which can cause stroke, seizures, mania, and psychosis.

In the United States, ephedrine, pseudoephedrine, and PPA are available over the counter for various uses. Preparations containing ephedrine are sold as bronchodilators for mild asthma. Both pseudoephedrine and PPA are ephedrine alkaloids found in many over-the-counter decongestant, cold, and allergy products, and PPA is found in weight-control products as well.

Co-Q-10

Coenzyme Q10 (or ubiquinone), usually referred to as Co-Q-10, is a fat-soluble compound synthesized by the body. It plays an essential role in converting food into energy and in protecting the body against damage from substances known as free radicals.

Co-Q-10 has shown promise in the treatment of obesity and candida (see Chapter 2). According to Melvyn Werbach, M.D., author of *Healing With Food,* there appears to be a relationship between the blood level of Co-Q-10 and obesity. Julian Whitaker, M.D., author of *Dr. Whitaker's Guide to Natural Healing,* reports that a deficiency of Co-Q-10 may contribute to deficient thermogenesis in people who are obese. Co-Q-10 also has gained much popularity in recent years as a defender against diseases caused by free-radical reactions, such as atherosclerosis, cancer, diabetes, and asthma, and in the prevention and treatment of heart disease.

The body's ability to produce its own supply of Co-Q-10 begins to decrease at around age 20. This decline has led many experts to recommend supplementation. Some health practitioners recommend a daily dose of 30 mg for healthy individuals and up to 150 mg a day for people who have heart disease, cancer, diabetes, or another medical condition. Dr. Werbach recommends 50 mg twice daily for obesity, while Dr. Whitaker suggests a similar amount: 20 to 30 mg three times daily. When taking Co-Q-10, be sure you are consuming enough vitamin E (400 to 800 IU, or international units), either in your diet or as a supplement, because vitamin E stimulates the natural production of Co-Q-10.

Paul Cheney, M.D., director of the Cheney Clinic in Charlotte, North Carolina, recommends taking sublingual Co-Q-10 lozenges instead of tablets, as the latter tend to be metabolized by the liver. Lozenges are not as readily available as tablets, so you may need to ask your pharmacist or physician for them.

DHEA

Dehydroepiandrosterone (DHEA) is produced by the adrenal gland and is the most abundant hormone in the human bloodstream. It is often touted as an anti-obesity "superhormone" because of its ability to metabolize fat and convert fat to muscle. It does this by blocking the action of an enzyme that is essential for fat production.

The level of DHEA in the human body peaks at about age 20, after which it decreases steadily. This decline has prompted some experts to recommend supplementation. DHEA is available over the counter in synthetic form or with animal extracts. At this time, there are no pure natural alternatives. However, the *Dioscorea villosa* plant, also known as the Mexican yam or wild yam, contains precursors (substances from which other substances are made) that some researchers say allow your body to easily produce its own DHEA. The suggested dosage of pure DHEA is 30 to 90 mg per day; follow package directions or those of your health care provider for both natural DHEA and wild yam supplements.

DHEA has been studied extensively and been the subject of countless studies in both animals and humans. In addition to its fat-fighting properties, DHEA is credited with slowing the aging process, combating cancer and heart disease, and boosting the immune system. Though DHEA appears to have many positive features, much is still not understood about it. Less serious side effects include acne, fatigue, irritability, oily skin, insomnia, and facial hair growth in some women. People with a personal or family history of any type of tumor that responds to hormones, such as breast or prostate cancer, should not take DHEA.

Omega-6 Fatty Acids

Omega-6 fatty acids are an essential part of a healthy diet. They play crucial roles in the production of prostaglandins, hormone-like substances that control all the organs in the body and regulate tissue function. Gammalinolenic acid (GLA) is an omega-6 fatty acid that is found in black currant oil, evening primrose oil, and borage oil. It is normally synthesized in the liver from linoleic acid that is present in the diet. People who consume large amounts of sugar, saturated fats from animal products, and trans fatty acids, however, typically have low levels of GLA.

GLA has been the subject of many studies, and results indicate that GLA may promote weight loss in people who have failed to lose weight despite appropriate diets. Difficulty in losing weight may be due to reduced brown fat activity, a process that is important when converting food into energy. Evening primrose oil appears to help normalize reduced brown fat activity. The people who seem to respond best to primrose oil are those with a family history of obesity.

Suggested daily doses of supplemental GLA are 500 to 1,500 mg of borage oil, 100 to 200 mg a day of black currant oil, and 500 to 1,500 mg of evening primrose oil. GLA supplementation also may help prevent cancer, kill existing cancer cells, help prevent clogging of arteries, reduce cholesterol levels, and reduce blood triglyceride levels.

Because a lower-fat diet often causes the body to increase its fat storage as a survival tactic, some nutritionists recommend supplementation with borage oil (one capsule two or three times a day) and flaxseed oil (1 teaspoon once a day) to help eliminate this tendency to stockpile fat.

Other Thermogenic Substances

There are many other single and combination thermogenic substances available on the market. Most of them can be found as additional ingredients in weight loss products that contain chromium and/or ephedra. The effectiveness of these other substances has not been proven in controlled studies, though they are probably safe. To help you know what you are buying and how it may affect you, descriptions of the most common additives are provided below.

• **Gugal.** This is a popular Indian Ayurvedic herb that contains compounds called guggulsterones. These substances increase the secretion of thyroid hormones in rats. This reaction may cause a rise in body temperature. Gugal is sold as a lone supplement as well as in combinations. Its value may be in helping to "kick-start" your metabolism rate if your morning body temperature is below the optimal range of 97.8 to 98.2 degrees. Take according to package directions.

• **Carnitine.** This nonessential (meaning the body has the ability to produce it) amino acid is required for optimal metabolism of fat, and for this reason some weight loss researchers suggest taking carnitine supplements. See Amino Acids in Chapter 6.

• **Yohimbine.** Yohimbine is the active component found in the bark of the yohimbé tree, which grows in West Africa. Yohimbine reportedly may stimulate the receptors that cause the body to hold on to fat. This benefit is questioned by many experts, who note that yohimbine has limited access to fat cells because there is poor blood flow in fat tissue.

Yohimbine must be used with caution. Do not use it if you are being treated for heart, kidney, thyroid, or psychiatric disease; high blood pressure; depression or anxiety; seizure disorders; stroke; or if you are taking antidepressants, MAO (monoamine oxidase) inhibitors, any prescription, or any products containing ephedrine or caffeine.

• **Pyruvate.** Pyruvate is a naturally occurring by-product of metabolism. Research on pyruvate indicates that supplementation may stimulate the metabolism and utilization of fat. In a University of Pittsburgh Medical Center study, obese women who took pyruvate daily while consuming 1,000 calories a day lost 37 percent more weight and 48 percent more fat than did women eating the same amount of calories but no pyruvate. Pyruvate may be useful in preventing the ''plateau'' that often occurs after several weeks of dieting. For that purpose, 20 grams per day for several days followed by a maintenance dose of 5 grams per day may be helpful.

• **Cayenne.** Despite its reputation as a hot herb, cayenne has a mild thermogenic effect. Among its primary functions is the promotion of blood flow and sweating to help eliminate wastes. Because of its stimulating abilities, it is added to thermogenic compounds primarily as a catalyst to help ensure that the other agents in the compound are effectively delivered. Cayenne can also be taken as a sole supplement, either in bulk or in capsules. Because cayenne is hot, use very little (about ⅛ teaspoon mixed into your food) at first and build up to ¼ teaspoon at each meal. If it is too hot for you, take capsules. Always take cayenne with food to prevent irritation to the stomach lining.

• **Guarana.** Guarana is a caffeine-containing herb that grows primarily in the Amazon jungle. An 800 mg dose of guarana is equivalent to 32 mg of caffeine. Guarana has been used for centuries by the Brazilian Indians and is commonly referred to as Brazilian cocoa. It is available commercially as a single supplement and in combination.

• **Garcinia cambogia.** This metabolism booster is found in the rind of the malabar tamarind, a fruit that grows in India. The rind contains hydroxycitric acid, which is the ingredient responsible for its weight control abilities. The hydroxycitric acid slows down the enzyme process that is responsible for producing fat in the body. The result of this process is an increase in thermogenesis. Results of animal studies also suggest that it may suppress appetite. Garcinia cambogia is available commercially as a single supplement and in combination products. As a single agent, a typical dose is 15 to 30 drops in 8 ounces of water, herbal tea, or fruit juice, taken one hour before meals. This reportedly helps to suppress appetite and satisfy food cravings. Garcinia cambogia is also available in tablets and can be taken at a dose of 500 mg three times a day.

The effectiveness of thermogenic substances in weight loss remains controversial for many researchers yet lauded by many individuals who use them. Until the two sides meet and answers are found, only you can decide if they are right for you. If not, perhaps you would like to explore the power of herbs and nutritional supplements in weight loss. We look at these substances next.

CHAPTER SIX

Herbs, Supplements, and Nutrients

Boosting your metabolic rate and burning fat are not the only ways to lose weight. Some natural substances can facilitate your weight loss efforts by suppressing your appetite or making you feel full, altering your mood, or encouraging evacuation of your kidneys and bowels. In this chapter we first look at some of the herbs that fulfill these tasks, including how they work, how to prepare your own weight loss remedies, and which herbal supplements are available on the market that can complement your weight loss efforts. In our discussion we look at the herbal forms of phen-fen, the dietary drug aid combination that was removed from the market in September 1997 by the FDA. One of the reported benefits of the herbal phen-fen combinations is increased metabolism of fat. Yet the other claims and the variety of herbs that may be contained in the different herbal forms of phen-fen on the market warrant its being discussed here rather than in the preceding chapter.

Other weight loss aids covered in this chapter include natural diuretics (for water weight), fiber products, and other weight control supplements. The products discussed are available from your pharmacy, herbalists, natural health physicians, or health food stores. Please consult with your health care provider before taking any herb, supplement, or nutrient.

Herbal Medicine for Weight Loss

Since ancient times, herbs have provided relief and healing to people around the world. Herbs contain dozens, sometimes hundreds, of active ingredients, such as vitamins, minerals, salts, enzymes, and proteins that work together to produce qualities that are unique for each plant. Though we don't know the exact reason why many herbs have positive effects on the body, we do know that, in general, the chemicals contained in plants can be easily metabolized by the human body. When you take an herb to treat a specific condition, its chemicals interact with the compounds in your body and address the purpose for which it was taken. Typically, you need to take herbs regularly for several days or weeks before you receive their full benefits.

One unique quality of herbs, which differentiates them from conventional drugs, is that they provide holistic healing: herbs deliver all of their components up for the healing process, and each of them works synergistically in the body. A drug, however, enters the body much like a foreign object, causing adverse effects and often creating imbalances.

Preparing Herbal Remedies
Herbal remedies can be prepared from the leaves, roots, bark, flowers, bulbs, stems, seeds, resin, fruit, or rhizomes of plants. Many of the herbs that can be used to support your weight loss and maintenance program can be purchased already prepared for you in the form of teas, tinctures, extracts, capsules, or powders, or you can purchase raw herbs and prepare your own remedies. You can get herbs from an

herbalist, at health or natural food stores, homeopathic pharmacies, or through a naturopath or mail-order house.

If you decide to prepare your own herbal remedies, the general instructions offered below can help you prepare infusions and decoctions (teas), extracts, and tinctures. Glass or earthenware pots are preferred over metal for preparing these formulas.

• **Infusions** are prepared like teas and are made from the leaves, flowers, or other soft parts of a plant. To prepare an infusion, pour 2 cups of boiling water over 2 to 3 tablespoons of the herb and steep in a glass or earthenware pot for at least 10 minutes or as long as recommended for the specific herb. Strain the liquid and drink the infusion hot, warm, or cool, depending on the herb. Herbal infusions decompose rapidly, so make a fresh batch daily and keep it refrigerated. Add lemon, fruit juice, or mint if the taste is a bit too unusual for you.

• **Decoctions** are also like teas, but they are prepared from the roots, stems, and bark of herbs. To prepare a standard decoction, boil 1 ounce of herb in 1 pint of water in a covered nonmetallic container for 20 to 30 minutes. Strain the liquid and let it cool. Decoctions also deteriorate rapidly and should be made fresh and kept refrigerated for no more than one or two days.

• **Extracts** are stronger than infusions and are readily available commercially. To make your own, the easiest preparation is a green extract made by thoroughly crushing the juicy parts of the plant and pressing out the juice. One ounce of extract equals 1 ounce of the pure dry herb. Extracts deteriorate rapidly, so make fresh batches as needed.

• **Tinctures** are a bit more time-consuming as they require six weeks to reach full potency. To prepare your own tincture, steep 1 ounce of dried herb in 5 ounces of vodka, gin, brandy, or grain alcohol or vinegar. Place in a tightly sealed dark glass container, mark the level on the outside of the container, and store it out of direct sunlight. Shake the container ten to one hundred times every day. If the tincture level goes down, add more of the original liquid to maintain the level. At six weeks, strain out the plant materials if you desire. Store the tincture in a cool, dark place.

Guidelines for Herbal Use

Herbs can be very potent and so should be used as directed and in moderation. Consider the following guidelines when using herbs.

➤ When used according to package directions or the advice of a knowledgeable practitioner, herbs are very safe. As with any substance, however, misuse or abuse may cause undesirable effects. An herbalist, naturopath, or homeopath can help you select herbs that are best for your system. Refer to Appendix A and the Suggested Readings in Appendix B for sources of information.

➤ Some herbs interact with prescription and over-the-counter drugs as well as with other herbs. If you are taking any conventional drug, including aspirin, insulin, or diabetic pills, consult with your physician or another professional who understands the pharmacology of both the herbs and your medications before you take an herbal remedy.

➤ Unless specifically instructed to do otherwise, take herbal remedies after you have eaten a meal or snack. Some herbs can cause nausea if you take them on an empty stomach.

➤ If you experience nausea, vomiting, diarrhea, or other unexpected symptoms after taking an herbal remedy, stop taking it and call your herbalist or physician. You may need to switch to a different herb.

Herbal Forms of Phen-Fen

The withdrawal from the market of the diet drug combination phen-fen (phentermine and fenfluramine) set the stage for a flurry of herbal alternatives to the drug-based dietary aid (phentermine alone remains on the market as a weight loss drug). The wording used to advertise these herbal products is, in most cases, careful to emphasize that the products are not dietary aids but herbal supplements designed to complement a weight reduction program that should include a nutritious, low-fat eating plan and exercise. Among the benefits of plant-based phen-fen products are that they help suppress the appetite, increase metabolic rate, improve energy level, help manage feelings of depression and anxiety associated with dieting, and reduce cholesterol levels.

The herbal alternatives to phen-fen each contain different ingredients, yet they all have St. John's Wort as their principal component. Cayenne, ephedra, garcinia, ginkgo, ginseng, gotu kola, hawthorn berry, kelp, and saw palmetto are some of the other ingredients you can expect to see on the label. Below we look at the role these herbs play in the herbal form of phen-fen.

Dosing

Herbal forms of phen-fen should be taken according to package directions. If you are pregnant, lactating, have high blood pressure, or are receiving treatment for a serious medical condition, consult with your physician before taking these supplements.

St. John's Wort

St. John's Wort has gained tremendous popularity both as an antidepressant and as an herbal supplement for weight loss. In ancient times it was widely used for diseases such as colds, tuberculosis, whooping cough, and syphilis, and as a folk remedy for depression, hysteria, insomnia, and fatigue.

This aromatic perennial herb got its name from the fact that the yellow flowers it produces seem to flourish on June 24, which is the traditional birthday of John the Baptist. The active ingredient in St. John's Wort is hypericin, which helps promote a calm feeling and a positive mental state. One explanation for the effectiveness of this herb in weight loss is that it eases the depression and anxiety often associated with trying to lose weight. It takes about two to four weeks for hypericin extract to develop its soothing effect, so don't expect immediate results.

The antidepressant effects of St. John's Wort have been linked to substances that inhibit monoamine oxidase. Certain foods should be avoided when taking St. John's Wort or any agent that inhibits monoamine oxidase. These include beer, wine, coffee, chocolate, yogurt, pickled or smoked foods, and fava beans. Also, if you have hypertension or are taking diet pills, cold or hay fever medications, amphetamines, nasal decongestants, tryptophan or tyrosine, narcotics, or asthma inhalants, check with your physician or pharmacist before taking St. John's Wort, as the combination may cause adverse effects.

Ephedra
Detailed information on this herb is in Chapter 5.

Saw Palmetto
The berries of saw palmetto *(Serenoa serrulata)* are believed to facilitate weight loss, although it is not understood how this occurs. Its ability to control weight gain was first observed by medical botanist John Lloyd, who noted that grazing farm animals fed saw palmetto berries grew up sleek and strong. This finding was verified later by medical researchers.

Garcinia

Garcinia cambogia. See details in Chapter 5.

Ginkgo

This most ancient of all living tree species has been supplying humankind with herbal remedies for more than 5,000 years. In the area of weight reduction, ginkgo *(Ginkgo biloba)* is responsible for enhancing the brain's metabolism of glucose, which in turn stimulates the weight reduction process. Ginkgo extracts have also been used to treat asthma, bronchitis, cardiovascular disease, senility, and hardening of the arteries. This herb is also rich in vitamin C, carotenoids, and compounds known collectively as ginkgolides, which have a powerful effect on increasing blood circulation and oxygen levels in the brain.

Cayenne

(Capsicum annum.) See Chapter 5 for details.

Gotu Kola

When combined with ginseng, gotu kola *(Centella asiatica)* can cause an increase in metabolic rate. Traditionally it is a diuretic and blood purifier that is used for diseases of the skin, nervous system, and blood. Gotu kola does not contain caffeine, and despite the similarity in names, has no association with kola nut.

Hawthorn Berry

The addition of hawthorn berry *(Crataegus oxyacantha)* to weight loss formulas is primarily to help decrease the stress placed on the heart and circulation by being overweight. It also helps tone up the heart muscle while you lose weight, especially if your weight reduction plan includes routine exercise.

Hawthorn is available as a single supplement; however,

that form is reserved for people who are using it to treat heart disease. The presence of hawthorn in a weight loss formula is all you need.

Kelp

Kelp (also called seaweed) appears to play several roles in weight loss. If you exercise regularly, seaweed can boost your body's ability to burn fat. Seaweed is also a good source of iodine. This nutrient is needed to maintain a healthy thyroid, the gland that controls metabolism. Kelp also acts as an appetite suppressant (see page 103) and lowers blood cholesterol levels.

Ginseng

Ginseng *(Panax schinseng)* stimulates the metabolism, reduces blood pressure, and protects the nervous system from stress. The value of ginseng in an herbal weight-loss supplement is that it allows the body to better cope with stress and tension by enabling it to normalize body functions. Ginseng is not a weight loss herb on its own.

Diuretics

Many women turn to diuretics for relief of temporary water-weight gain associated with premenstrual syndrome and the menstrual cycle. Diuretics are also effective in reducing lymphatic swelling and in weight loss. Herbalists from around the world have used various plants for their natural diuretic properties for centuries, and now many of these single and compound remedies are available on pharmacy and natural food store shelves. When taking diuretics, you may need to take a potassium supplement (200–500 mg/day) to prevent depletion of your potassium. The body loses much of its potassium reserves during excess urination.

Some of the more popular herbs used as diuretics are

listed below. Which one you choose is a matter of personal taste, availability, and preference for any additional properties the herb may offer.

• **Dandelion** *(Taraxacum officinale):* You may take a second look at this "weed" once you discover how versatile it can be. The dandelion's diuretic properties were discovered in the tenth century by Arab physicians, and it is still used for this purpose today. This herb is also valued for its high content of vitamins A and C, for its assistance in digesting fats, and for its treatment of liver and kidney disorders and vaginal yeast infections.

Dandelions are a low-calorie herb/food that can be consumed in a number of ways. The young leaves can be used in salads, while the larger leaves can be eaten steamed. The roots can be dried and ground into a powder to use as a coffee substitute and for its diuretic abilities.

To prepare a decoction, boil 2 to 3 teaspoons of powdered root in one cup of water for 15 minutes. Let it cool. If you prefer to use the leaves, place ½ teaspoon of dried leaves in a cup of boiling water and let it steep for 15 minutes. Take up to three cups a day of either preparation.

• **Parsley Root** *(Petroselinum* spp.): Parsley is also useful as a digestive aid. Dose: If making an infusion with the leaves, use 1 ounce per pint of water and drink three cups per day. If using the root, prepare a decoction and prepare the same as infusion.

• **Uva-Ursi** *(Arctostaphylos uva-ursi):* This herb contains tannins, which act as a diuretic. If you prepare infusions of this herb, do not boil the herb, because this destroys its healing properties. Instead, boil 1 pint of water and let it cool slightly before pouring it over 1 ounce of the herb. Let it steep for 15 minutes. Drink three cups a day at room temperature or cooler. If you prefer to use the tincture, add 10 to 30 drops into a glass of water and take up to three times a day.

• **Corn Silk** *(Zea mays):* The fine, soft threads of female corn plants are known as corn silk. This mildly sweet herb has been used for centuries by various North and Central American Indian societies as a diuretic and to treat urinary problems. Today those traditional uses have extended well beyond the Indian culture.

The presence of tannins in corn silk is responsible for its diuretic properties. To prepare an infusion, use 2 ounces of herb per 16 ounces of boiling water. Allow to steep for 15 to 20 minutes and drink two to three cups per day.

• **Juniper Berries** *(Juniperus communis):* This herb is often combined with uva-ursi to help lose water weight. As a diuretic, juniper may also help reduce bloating associated with menstruation. Juniper also has anti-inflammatory properties and is useful in relieving the pain of arthritis. Because juniper can stimulate uterine contractions, it should not be used by pregnant women.

To prepare an infusion, use 1 ounce of bruised berries per pint of boiling water. Let it steep 10 to 20 minutes. Drink up to two cups a day for no longer than six weeks. Large doses of juniper can cause kidney damage, and people with kidney problems should not use juniper.

Herbal Appetite Suppressants

Several herbs can be used to help curb appetite and reduce food cravings.

• **Spirulina:** This ultra-high-protein plant food is often touted as an effective appetite suppressant because it contains the amino acid phenylalanine. This claim is denied by some researchers (see Phenylalanine, page 107). Spirulina is also credited with the ability to stimulate metabolism, suppress fatty accumulations in the liver, and reduce total cholesterol levels. The usual dosage is 1 to 2 tablespoons per day, dissolved in water or other beverage.

Spirulina belongs to a group of foods known as "green foods" because of its high concentration of chlorophyll. Other common green foods include alfalfa, wheat grass, blue-green algae (which contain the appetite suppressant phenylalanine), and kelp (also called seaweed; see below).

• **Seaweed** *(Fucus vesiculosus):* This herb from the sea curbs appetite and has diuretic properties. To prepare an infusion, steep 1 heaping teaspoon of dried seaweed in 8 ounces of hot water for 30 minutes. Drink three to four cups a day one hour before meals and one before retiring.

• **Chickweed** *(Stelleria media):* Chickweed is one of the most common weeds and is an old wives' remedy for obesity. It is reportedly beneficial as an appetite suppressant, diuretic, and laxative. To prepare an infusion, use 1 ounce of dried herb per 16 ounces of boiling water. Let steep 15–20 minutes. Drink three cups or more per day. If you use the extract, the daily dose is 10 to 60 drops added to water. Chickweed is also a nutritious food. The young leaves, when boiled, taste much like spinach and are rich in vitamins and minerals yet low in calories.

• **Fennel** *(Foeniculum vulgare):* This native to the Mediterranean area has been associated with weight loss and appetite suppression since medieval times. Fennel seeds were chewed by people in medieval Europe and by the Puritans in America during religious fasts to ward off hunger. It is also a mild diuretic. This herb is available in powder form and capsules. Follow package directions.

• **Plantain** *(Plantago ovata;* also *P. major* and *P. lanceolata):* The *P. ovata* variety is recommended by Dr. Daniel Mowrey, author of *The Scientific Validation of Herbal Medicine,* because of its "appetite-satiating" effect and its ability to reduce fat absorption. The species *P. major* and *P. lanceolata* have diuretic properties.

In June 1997, the FDA issued a warning to consumers about the use of any dietary supplements, including teas, that listed plantain as an ingredient. The concern centered around the fact that some of these products were mislabeled and actually contain digitalis, a powerful heart stimulant that can cause cardiac arrest and other life-threatening heart problems. Digitalis can also cause nausea, vomiting, dizziness, confusion, low blood pressure, headache, and vision problems. (The plantain in question is the herb and not the banana-like fruit found in some grocery stores.)

The FDA urges consumers to check the labels of any dietary supplements for plantain and to get an update on the companies and products that may contain digitalis by calling the FDA's Consumer Hotline at 1-800-FDA-4010 or accessing their website (http://vm.cfsan.fda.gov/~dms/supplmnt.html).

Growth Hormone

The use of growth hormone or natural products that promote the release of growth hormone to lose weight deserves mention, as some researchers believe people can lose weight by increasing the natural output of growth hormone by the pituitary gland. Some scientists believe supplementation becomes important after age 30, when there is a sharp decline in the production and release of natural growth hormone.

Growth hormone is a polypeptide that is released into the bloodstream by the pituitary gland. Growth hormone increases fat loss by releasing stockpiled body fat and sending it into the bloodstream as free fatty acids, which your body can burn for energy. Release can be stimulated by exercise, stress, trauma, sleep, hypoglycemia, fasting, and amino acid stimulation. One way to do this is to take an amino acid combination that contains *arginine pyroglutamate* and *lysine*. The suggested dosage for weight loss and for stimulating growth hormone production is 500 mg twice daily of each amino acid, or 1,000 to 1,500 mg of each taken before bed. (See Amino Acids, below.) The use of both growth hormones and the amino acids arginine and lysine to promote their production is controversial and unproven. Supplements of arginine exceeding 30 mg daily should be avoided by anyone with a history of schizophrenia.

Amino Acids

Use of amino acids is another controversial area in weight loss and control. Amino acids are proteins that the body either produces (nonessential amino acids) or must get from food (essential). Some health professionals believe that, if used properly, amino acids can be very helpful in controlling appetite and metabolizing fat deposits. Others warn that the potential for misuse is too great and their use should be discouraged.

Generally, health professionals agree that use of individual amino acids can cause an imbalance of overall amino acid levels in the body. Therefore, amino acid supplementation needs to be monitored closely and should not exceed several weeks in duration. For people who want to take an amino acid supplement, some experts suggest they take a general one separate from and in addition to any individual amino acid to ensure against any deficiencies.

Carnitine

Carnitine is a nonessential amino acid that is produced in the liver and converted from lysine and methionine (two other nonessential amino acids). It has a significant role in the metabolism of fat, may reduce feelings of hunger, and helps keep triglyceride levels low. Carnitine requires adequate levels of vitamin C in order to metabolize fats effectively. A typical dosage is 1 to 3 grams per day. If you take carnitine, a 500 to 1,000 mg supplement of vitamin C is suggested if you do not get enough vitamin C from your food.

Methionine

Methionine is an essential amino acid that, when used for weight control, is usually taken in a supplement combination consisting of phenylalanine, tryptophan, valine, and methionine. This supplement can significantly reduce appetite among people who are overweight but does not appear to have the same effect on people of normal weight. It is believed this reduction occurs because the amino acids stimulate a hormone that signals the brain that enough food has been consumed to satisfy hunger. The suggested dosage of the combination supplement is 3 grams phenylalanine, 2 grams each valine and methionine, and 1 gram tryptophan, taken once daily before a meal. Methionine is also valued as a detoxifying aid for helping eliminate heavy metals from the body.

Phenylalanine

This nonessential amino acid may curb your appetite by increasing the brain's production of the neurotransmitters dopamine and norepinephrine. These two neurotransmitters, along with a third called acetylcholine, are involved in appetite control.

The chemical structure of phenylalanine is similar to that of the over-the-counter appetite depressant phenylpropanolamine (PPA), which is found in products such as Dexatrim. Proponents of phenylalanine as an appetite suppressant explain that it differs from PPA because the artificial drug causes the brain to use up its supply of norepinephrine. Once a person's supply of norepinephrine is depleted, which can take as little as a few days, he or she usually goes on a rebound eating binge. Use of the natural amino acid phenylalanine does not cause this reaction because it is a natural nutrient the brain can use to make more of the neurotransmitter.

The experts do not agree on when to take phenylalanine or whether it is safe or beneficial as an appetite suppressant. Pharmacognosist Varro Tyler, Ph.D., author of *The Honest Herbal,* says that "there's no evidence phenylalanine is effective in reducing the appetite." Some researchers suggest taking between 100 and 500 mg before a meal; others recommend taking it on an empty stomach before retiring. In either case, phenylalanine should not be used for longer than three weeks without a break or close medical supervision. Phenylalanine supplements are dangerous to pregnant or nursing women, growing children, people who are taking MAO inhibitors, and anyone with diabetes, high blood pressure, or melanoma skin cancer. If your overall protein intake is low, taking phenylalanine supplements may cause an amino acid imbalance and the possibility of depression and eye lesions. Given the availability of other, safer products for appetite suppression, phenylalanine is probably best avoided.

Valine

This essential amino acid is found in soy flour, brown rice, almonds, brazil nuts, lentils, chickpeas, raw lima beans, and mushrooms. Valine should be taken in a supplement combination consisting of phenylalanine, tryptophan, and methionine. This supplement can significantly reduce appetite among people who are overweight but does not appear to have the same effect on people of normal weight. It is believed this reduction occurs because the amino acids stimulate a hormone that signals the brain that enough food has been consumed to satisfy hunger. The suggested dosage of the combination supplement is 3 grams phenylalanine, 2 grams each valine and methionine, and 1 gram tryptophan, taken once daily before a meal.

Digestive Aids for Weight Loss

Support of the digestive system is essential as it improves the utilization of nutrients, promotes proper food metabolism, and reduces cravings and the desire to overeat.

• One quick and easy digestive aid to prepare is *lemon water*. Squeeze half a small lemon into 8 ounces of water and drink it 15 to 30 minutes before your meals. This helps in the digestion and utilization of fats.

• Another quick digestive aid consists of 1 tablespoon of pure *apple-cider vinegar* in one 8-ounce glass of water. Drink during your meal. The vinegar contains potassium, which can break up and dissolve fats. (To prevent erosion of tooth enamel, drink this mixture through a straw.)

• *Liquid chlorophyll* is another excellent digestive system supporter. A teaspoon or two added to water or to a diluted fruit or tomato juice twice daily helps to nourish the stomach lining and improve digestion. When your food is assimilated better, you are less likely to have food cravings.

• If your physician has told you that you have an enzyme deficiency, you can add *digestive enzymes* to your diet to help eliminate food cravings. Enzymes work with the body, not against it. When you eliminate food cravings, it becomes more possible to adopt healthy eating habits.

There are several ways to increase your intake of digestive enzymes. One way is to eat plenty of uncooked, unprocessed, organically grown (preferred) food. Some health professionals recommend you eat raw food both before and after you eat a meal; say, a carrot before and parsley or fresh fruit after. This puts the enzymes right to work. Juicing fruits and vegetables offers enzymes in a glass, although it does remove the fiber. When cooking foods, choose low-heat, slow-cooking methods and go very light on the salt.

You can also add specific enzyme supplements to your diet, either by prescription or over the counter. Two popular and effective enzymes are bromelain and papain, which are derived from the pineapple and papaya, respectively. Take two to three digestive enzyme tablets after meals. If you do not have the supplements, eat either papaya or pineapple after your meals for their digestive enzyme properties.

Hormone Balancing

Women who have an excess of estrogen in their system as compared with progesterone levels will have trouble losing weight, says Hunter Yost, M.D. High estrogen levels cause bloating, swelling, and difficulty with weight loss. The addition of progesterone can balance out the excess estrogen. Women who apply a progesterone cream to the abdominal area daily during the second half of their menstrual cycle can expect great relief from symptoms of premenstrual syndrome such as weight gain.

Fiber

The importance of sufficient fiber in the diet has already been mentioned in Chapter 3. If you are not getting at least 25 grams of fiber a day from your food, you need to add more fiber to your diet. There are several good supplemental sources available in pharmacies and health food stores. Fiber supplements are available in pills, raw bran, oat bran, capsules, and drinks.

Supplementing your diet with natural fibers can help you stay on course with your new eating plan, because they make you feel full. They also stabilize the absorption of carbohydrates and thus help even out blood glucose levels. When taking fiber supplements, make sure you drink at least eight glasses of water a day; ten is preferred. Here are several fiber supplements for you to consider.

• **Psyllium** is a natural laxative that is rich in soluble fiber. When added to the diet, it can decrease appetite, soften stools naturally and make it easier for the colon to pass and eliminate them, and help reduce fat absorption by coating the intestines. Psyllium, which is the seed of the fleawort plant, can be purchased as whole seeds or ground to a powder, and it is available as the primary ingredient in many over-the-counter laxatives. It is available in several commercial brands or in bulk. It is also used as a cholesterol-lowering agent and to help reduce the risk of cancer of the rectum or colon.

For people with high cholesterol levels, many medical experts recommend taking psyllium daily to bring those levels down. The addition of psyllium to the diet can also reduce the risk of cancer of the colon or rectum.

Because psyllium forms an indigestible mass when ingested, do not take it with any other supplements or medications. If taking raw psyllium, stir $1/2$ to 1 teaspoon of the husks in 8 ounces of water and drink the entire glass. Take twice a day. Follow the package directions on any commercial brands.

• **Pectin** is derived from apple pulp and the rinds of oranges and lemons after they have been squeezed for their juice. It reduces appetite, absorbs water, and decreases the amount of fat absorption. Take according to package directions.

• **Guar gum** is a soluble fiber that comes from the guar plant in the Middle East. It helps hinder fat absorption from the intestines and also slows glucose uptake in the intestines, making it useful in treating diabetes. Take according to package directions.

You may see other fiber products on the market that list ingredients in addition to those mentioned above. Some of those ingredients may include vegetable and citrus fiber, uva-ursi, shave grass, corn silk and watermelon seed, chickweed, licorice root, saffron flowers, gotu kola, kelp, echinacea root, black walnut hulls, fennel seed, dandelion root, hawthorn berries, and papaya leaves.

Special Needs

Management of Candida

Presence of the yeast *Candida albicans* in your system can contribute to weight gain by making your body store fat, especially among both young and postmenopausal women. Natural therapies to decrease the amount of yeast in the intestinal tract include caprylic acid, garlic, and the herb pau d'arco. Caprylic acid is extracted from coconut oil and is a natural fatty acid. Although it does not always kill the yeast, it significantly reduces the population. It must be taken for up to four months, depending on the severity of infection. Recommended starting dose is 300 to 600 mg per day, working up to 1,300 to 2,000 mg three times a day with meals.

Garlic contains two antifungal agents, allin and haconi, which are effective against candida. A daily garlic regimen of four to six capsules of garlic oil or garlic extract often kills yeast. It is not recommended if you have low blood pressure, however. Pau d'arco, which is derived from a Brazilian tree bark, is another effective antifungal agent. It is available in capsules or as a tea. Take two to four capsules or two cups of tea per day. Another remedy is a formula called Candacin, which contains grapefruit seed extract, black walnut, goldenseal, and bearberry leaf.

Once one has had candidiasis, it is necessary to restore the natural state of the colon by reintroducing healthy bacteria, including *Lactobacillus acidophilus, L. bifidus,* and *Streptococcus faecium*. These are available in several products, including Vital-Plex and DDS-1. Other ways to revitalize the intestinal flora include taking 1 to 2 tablets of hydrochloric acid with meals and 2 to 3 digestive enzyme tablets after meals.

Cleansing the Lymphatic System

A well-functioning lymphatic system is necessary for effective metabolism. To help cleanse the lymph system, you can take 2 capsules of echinacea, three times a day, or 10 to 20 drops of tincture three times a day. This herb, which is native to North America, is also an important therapeutic plant for boosting the immune system. (Also see Chapter 1, Sluggish Lymphatic System.)

Detoxifying the Liver

A toxic liver can make it difficult to lose weight (see Chapter 1, Toxic Liver). To help restore, support, and detoxify the liver, you can use the following approach for a liver flush. Consult with your physician before trying this treatment.

For three days, eat only organic apples and drink only organic apple juice and pure water. On the third day, mix together ¼ cup of extra-virgin olive oil and ¼ cup freshly squeezed lemon juice. To this you may add 1 tablespoon of disodium phosphate, but only under the guidance of your physician. After drinking the mixture, lie on your right side with your knees drawn up near your chest. Stay in this position for about 30 minutes. You may experience some mild cramping. This detoxification method works on both the liver and gallbladder. Within a few hours of drinking the mixture, you will likely eliminate bowel material that is green (bile) and contains particles that resemble gravel and sand.

All of the supplements and techniques discussed in this chapter can serve as complements to your weight loss efforts. Any one or more of them may be the catalyst you need to get you started or past a plateau in your program.

CHAPTER SEVEN

"Sensing" Weight Loss: Touch and Smell

Now we move away from food and look—and poke and press—at your body. Did you know you can massage your metabolism into high gear, poke food cravings away, or press the soles of your feet to suppress your appetite? All of these things, and more, are possible when you use acupuncture, acupressure, massage, and reflexology as part of your weight loss and maintenance program. In this chapter you can discover how to suppress your hunger, promote fat metabolism, and eliminate toxins from the body, either alone or with the help of professional therapists, using these body therapy techniques. Or you can let your nose help you lose weight. Certain aromas can regulate or decrease the desire for food. That's because there is a physiological connection between the satiety center in the brain and the odor of food. Therefore, we look at how aromatherapy can be a weight loss aid.

Acupuncture

Are you willing to have needles stuck into your outer ear to curb your appetite and reduce your sugar cravings? Thousands of people do it every day. They report that acupuncture is the extra help they need, along with a healthy eating plan and exercise, to lose weight and keep it off.

Although acupuncture is an ancient healing art perfected by the Chinese, it was a French physician, Dr. Nogier, who in 1957 discovered that ear (or auricular) acupuncture is effective in the treatment of obesity. Its success is due to the accessibility of the nerves and the ease of treatment. Acupuncturists can insert a small needle or staple in your outer ear and leave it in for hours or days with little worry that it will be jarred loose. When you feel hungry or have a craving for sweets, you can press on the staple for a minute or two to alleviate the desire to eat.

About 80 percent of people who undergo ear acupuncture for weight problems report reduced appetite, a feeling of fullness, and changes in their taste. The most common taste change is that less spicy foods become tastier, and these foods usually contain less salt, less fat, and fewer calories. For reasons not yet understood, many people who experience ear acupuncture also report a decline in total cholesterol and triglyceride levels. Other benefits associated with ear acupuncture include improvement in irritable colon and stomach problems, and better sleep and mood.

Although most people who use acupuncture report positive effects, only those who reduce caloric intake and increase energy consumption lose body weight. Individuals who rely on acupuncture needles alone hardly ever lose weight or reduce their risk factors for disease.

Acupressure

Acupressure is an ancient Chinese healing technique in which you, or an acupuncture practitioner, apply pressure, usually with the fingers or hands, to specific acupoints on the body as a way to restore the flow of energy, or *chi,* as it is referred to in Chinese culture. Energy becomes blocked in the body at sites that have been injured by physical trauma or constricted by tension and stress. Application of acupressure releases bottled-up energy and allows free flow of energy, facilitates weight loss by stimulating your metabolism to help you eliminate excess water, suppresses your appetite, improves circulation of lymph and blood, permits better elimination of toxins from the body, and relieves stress.

Both acupressure and acupuncture (see above) are based on Eastern teachings which say that a vital flow of energy moves throughout the body along twelve channels called *meridians*. Each meridian is associated with a different body system, yet they are all interconnected. At various sites along the meridians are acupoints where the meridians reach the skin surface. Each point is associated with a specific organ system, gland, or function. When you apply pressure to any of these points, your energy flow can be manipulated and balanced.

Acupressure for Overweight

The acupressure treatment explained below incorporates acupoints that can aid digestion, facilitate elimination of toxins, stimulate the metabolism, and reduce water retention. If you have an opportunity to experience a full-body acupressure session, we recommend it as a way to help place your entire body in balance. A full-body session is best done by a professional acupressure therapist or a friend or spouse who can learn the basic techniques in several hours from a licensed professional or from an illustrated book (see *Basic*

Shiatsu by Michio Kushi and other books in Appendix B). You also can self-treat with acupressure, although a few points may be hard or impossible to reach. We suggest you learn the technique from a trained, licensed professional so you can learn firsthand which points to treat, how much pressure to apply, and how a treatment feels.

Specific Trigger Points for Weight Loss

Figure 7–1 shows the acupoints discussed in the acupressure routine described below. Sit in a comfortable chair or recline on a firm, comfortable surface. At each acupoint, use your thumb or index finger and apply light and then increasingly more pressure to each site. The amount of pressure should produce a "good hurt." Hold the pressure for at least 10 seconds and then massage the point by slowly rotating your thumb or finger in a tight circular motion for one minute or longer.

• Begin with the Spleen meridian, which runs along the inside of the leg. Apply pressure and massage all the Spleen acupoints, paying particular attention to SP9 (inside of the leg below the knee and under the large bone), which helps relieve water retention, varicose veins, knee problems, and leg tension; SP6, located four finger-widths above the ankle, relieves water retention. *Do not* stimulate this point if you are pregnant.

• Move your hands to your rib cage and place your thumbs underneath at CV14. As you exhale, gently press inward and upward on CV14 and then go on to LV14, GB24, and LV13. These points are on both sides of the body, and you can treat both sides simultaneously. This acupressure sequence stimulates the liver, pancreas, stomach, and spleen. Repeat the sequence several times.

• Below the rib cage, locate CV6, which is three finger-

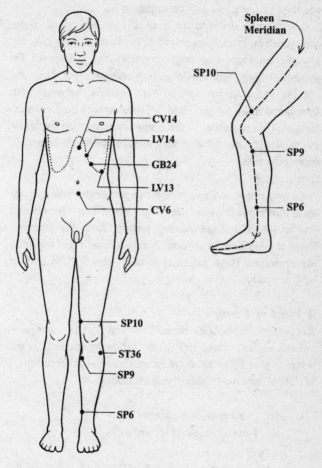

Figure 7-1.

widths directly below your belly button. Pressure on this acupoint relieves gas and constipation.

• Now move down to the front of your legs to the Stomach meridian. Locate acupoint ST36—four finger-widths below the kneecap, one finger-width to the outside of the shinbone. This point aids digestion and intestinal function.

• Press the fleshy part of your earlobe between your thumb and index finger. Hold 8–10 seconds to help suppress hunger. This is similar to the acupuncture method explained on page 116, though the acupuncture approach is usually more effective.

As you press and massage these acupoints, you help release blockages in your energy flow. Once they are released, you will feel a slight pulsing coming from the acupoint. Often it takes several sessions before you will feel this pulsing sensation. Have patience; it takes time for the body to heal naturally.

A Word of Caution

Acupressure stimulates blood flow and can be harmful to individuals who have any of the following medical conditions. If you go to an acupressure therapist, inform him or her about any medications you are taking.

• Fever or a contagious disease
• Risk of hemorrhage or thrombosis
• Osteoporosis
• Recent tissue damage, bone fractures, or inflammation. Avoid acupressure in the affected areas.
• Pregnancy. Some pressure points on the leg may increase the chance of miscarriage.
• High blood pressure or epilepsy.

Reflexology

Reflexology involves pressing and massaging specific reflex sites on the feet, hands, and ears that can help you curb your appetite and eliminate food cravings. If reflexology sounds similar to acupressure, you are right: they both make use of similar points for treatment. A major difference between the two is this: In acupressure, the points relate to specific body locations in relation to the meridians; in reflexology, the points correspond to nerve endings via nerve pathways. Application of pressure to reflex points can help suppress hunger and stimulate the function of certain glands and organs to help the body lose fat.

Reflexology for Weight Loss

Reflex points that are effective for weight loss and appetite suppression are associated with the endocrine glands and the colon, kidneys, and liver. We begin with a point that suppresses appetite. It is located just above the center of the lip between the nose and the edge of the lip (see Figure 7–2a). When you press on this point, you open up the message pathway to the brain to suppress appetite. Use a rotating motion for 8 to 10 seconds on this point.

A set of reflex points on the ear also can be pressed for appetite suppression. First, insert the tip of your index fingers gently into your ears with your palms facing toward your cheeks. Then use your thumb to press on the site that is between the reflex points for the forehead and the back of the head (see Figure 7–2b). With the reflex point between your index finger and thumb, squeeze it for one minute or more. Then use your third finger to press on the small indentation just in front of and just slightly above the tragus point. Work this reflex point for a minute or more as well.

Take a minute or two to work any or all of these reflex

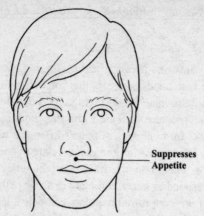

**Suppresses
Appetite**

Figure 7–2a

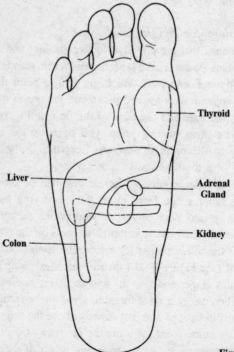

Thyroid

Liver

Adrenal
Gland

Kidney

Colon

Figure 7–2c

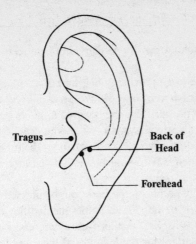

Figure 7–2b

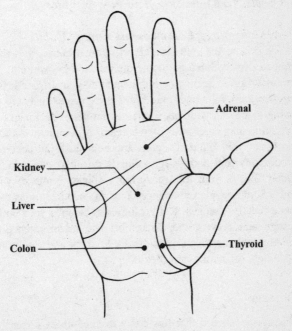

Figure 7–2d

points throughout the day to help eliminate feelings of hunger.

Experts believe reflexology helps repress hunger by affecting the vagus nerve, one of five cranial nerves that send messages to the ear. The vagus nerve involves the workings of the gastrointestinal system. When you press on the reflex points named on page 121, it normalizes the hunger signals that are on their way to your brain, and you lose much or all of your hunger pangs.

Other reflex points on the body can be pressed to help the body rid itself of fat. These points involve the adrenal and thyroid glands as well as the liver, colon, and kidneys. See Figure 7–2c and d for the location of these sites on the feet and hands. Take time to work them several times a day.

How Reflexology Complements Eating Habits

In addition to the reflex points mentioned above, you may want to explore having a complete reflexology workout. As you incorporate healthy eating habits into your life, reflexology can help your body maximize the changes that will be taking place. As your body releases fat reserves, for example, some may enter your bloodstream. A complete workout can boost your internal organs and help flush out accumulated toxins your body is releasing. Reflexology can help the added fiber in your diet move more efficiently out of your body. Some people experience bouts of constipation as they make dietary changes. Reflexology can balance your entire system and prevent the discomfort and inconvenience of bowel problems. See Appendix B, Sources and Suggested Readings, for books on reflexology.

Massage

Massage is a word that has come to encompass dozens of types of hands-on therapy that involve working on the soft tissues of the body. The word itself is from the Greek word *massein,* which means "to knead," although kneading is just one of several massage strokes that are used.

When it is used in conjunction with an exercise program, the place of massage in weight loss is to facilitate fat loss, promote muscle tone, and help eliminate toxins from the body. Not only does it complement weight loss; it also can help improve your mood and help you feel better about your body, which can in turn encourage you to stay on track with your weight loss efforts.

You can do self-massage or have a spouse or friend do it for you. It is preferable to work with someone as it allows your muscles to relax more fully, and your partner can massage places you may not be able to reach.

Below are some simple massage tips for weight loss. They incorporate several basic massage strokes and are written for a partner to give the massage to you. To promote weight loss, massage focuses on the fleshy areas, such as the sides of the abdomen, the buttocks, and thighs. A full-body massage, however, can help improve circulation and lymph flow throughout your entire body as well as make you feel completely relaxed. See Appendix A to help you find a massage therapist. Or you and a friend may want to take a massage course and learn how to give a massage to each other.

• *Kneading* is done on areas that have no bone immediately between the soft tissue, which makes it an excellent stroke to use for weight loss. To knead, place both hands next to each other over the site to be massaged. Keep your fingers straight as you pick up the flesh in one hand and pass it over to the other hand, as if you were kneading dough. This technique can be used on the sides of the abdomen, the thighs, and the buttocks.

• *Hacking* is done on large muscles, such as those in the thighs and back. Hold your fingers together and turn your hands horizontal to the site to be massaged. Keep your hands relaxed and your wrists loose as you bring each hand up and down quickly on the skin in a chopping motion. To determine how much force to use, practice on your own thigh first.

Stimulation of the Lymph System

To help stimulate a sluggish lymphatic system (see Chapter 1), you can visit a professional who does lymphatic therapy, or you can easily and safely stimulate your own lymph system with massage. Using a gentle, light touch, massage the drainage points of the lymphatic system, which are located at the small depression at the base of the throat and at the nodes in the groin, knees, and underarms. In addition to massage, you can raise your arms over your head for a few minutes every day, which can help open axillary (underarm) nodes. Also, sitting with your feet elevated is good for drainage from the legs into groin-area nodes.

A total-body skin massage using a skin brush is another way to promote healthy movement of lymphatic fluid throughout the body. One session of dry skin-brushing is said to be equivalent to twenty minutes of exercise. If possible, plan your skin-brushing session before your bath or shower.

Use a long-handled natural-bristle skin brush, available in pharmacies and natural food stores. Start with short strokes, moving from your fingertips up the inner and outer surfaces of each arm toward the heart. Use light, brisk strokes that cause tingling and flush the skin pink but do not irritate the skin. Once the arms are completed, move to your feet and use the same short strokes to brush upward toward the heart, one leg at a time. Include the top and the sole of each foot, the front and back of the legs, the pelvis, the abdomen, the buttocks, and the lower back. Avoid the head, neck, and chest areas.

Aromatherapy

Aromatherapy is the therapeutic use of the fragrances of plants' essential oils. Essential oils are the highly concentrated aromatic substances that are stored in glands in various parts of plants. They are pressed out of the plant parts and stored in glass bottles in their concentrated form until ready for use. Essential oils are inhaled from the container, added to a bath, or mixed with a carrier oil and applied to the skin as a massage or compress.

Essential oils affect the body in two ways: through sense of smell (olfactory) and absorption through the skin. When the vapors are inhaled, they directly affect various parts of the brain. When using aromatherapy for weight loss, essential oils are chosen that affect the satiety center of the brain. When the oils are absorbed through the skin, they reach the bloodstream and lymph system in about twenty minutes. From the bloodstream the oils branch out to all parts of the body.

Below are two aromatherapy blends that can help suppress appetite. The first is an inhalant you can carry with you. The second is a massage oil you can apply to your abdomen. Use either formula whenever you feel the urge to eat between meals or to overeat. See the box Guidelines for Using Essential Oils, page 128.

- Combine 15 drops of bergamot oil and 10 drops of fennel oil in a glass bottle that has an airtight cover. Gently roll the bottle between your palms until the oils are mixed. Use as an inhalant.
- Blend the following ingredients: ½ ounce carrier oil, 10 drops fennel oil, 5 drops bergamot oil, and 3 drops patchouli oil. Apply the formula to your abdominal area several times a day, as needed. If your skin will be exposed to the sun,

eliminate the bergamot oil from the formula, as it increases sensitivity to the sun.

Guidelines for Using Essential Oils

•Essential oils are very concentrated and must be diluted before you apply them to your skin. For this purpose use a carrier oil such as jojoba, almond, apricot kernel, canola, or sunflower oil.

• When using essential oils, always recap the bottles immediately.

• Use only glass containers, preferably ones with droppers. If it's necessary to use plastic, always add the carrier oil to the container first before adding the essential oils.

• Never shake essential formulas to mix them. Rather, roll the bottle gently between your palms or turn the bottle over several times.

• More is not better. Never add more than the stated amount of drops to a formula. You can, however, add less.

A novel approach to using aromas for weight loss has been developed by Alan R. Hirsch, M.D., whose research at the Smell and Taste Treatment and Research Foundation, Ltd., in Chicago, shows that certain odors have a direct suppressive effect on the ventromedial nucleus of the hypothalamus, a fancy name for the satiety center of the brain. Dr. Hirsch developed an inhaler that releases a specific manufactured odor that reportedly reduces the urge to overeat or to give in to cravings. In his study, the results of which were published in *Journal of Neurological and Orthopedic Medicine and Surgery* (1995), more than 3,000 study participants inhaled peppermint, banana, and green apple odors from an inhaler whenever they felt hungry. Individuals who responded best to the inhalers lost an average of 4.7 pounds per month during the six-month study. Characteristics that correlated with weight loss included frequency of inhaler use, having a medium or large frame, liking chocolate, and possessing good olfactory (sense of smell) abilities. People who have asthma or who experience migraine headaches should not use these inhalers. (See Appendix A for additional sources of information.)

Of the many interesting findings that emerged from Dr. Hirsch's research is the recommendation that people who want to lose weight should not eat dairy products. Infants need milk, and a mother's milk supply is determined by the amount her infant consumes. Yet milk and milk products are bland and do not trigger the satiety center in the brain. Many adults find they can eat large amounts of ice cream or cheese without feeling full. This is because the satiety center is not triggered by a milk odor. Thus, Dr. Hirsch recommends that anyone who wants to lose weight and keep it off should avoid dairy products, including low-fat and no-fat selections.

This chapter has demonstrated how you can utilize some very simple and accessible tools—your hands and your nose—and perhaps a needle or two to help you lose weight. We urge you to try these approaches and see how they work for you. What have you got to lose? Pounds!

CHAPTER EIGHT

Mind over (Food) Matter: Stress Reduction

Your mother-in-law is coming to live with you. You need to take a second job to pay the bills. Your car broke down on the freeway. The one-hour commute to work and back each day is affecting your attitude at work and at home. Your dog has fleas, and now so does your house. You have no time to study for exams in between working and going to school. Your spouse just lost his job. You're worried about your kids, who are seeing the wrong friends.

Life's stressors, big and small, day after day, are the fuel that drive many overweight people to the kitchen and fast-food counter. Most of the reasons people overeat or have poor eating habits are associated with how well they handle the stress or emotional turmoil in their lives. Stress triggers a psychological yearning and hunger for food . . . and that desire is for food that is fattening. Think about the last time you ate in response to a stressful situation or feeling: Did you reach for celery sticks or a bag of corn chips? A bowl of steamed veggies or a box of cookies? Even if you did force yourself to crunch a few carrots, you didn't feel satisfied and soon you were reaching for what you really wanted: ice cream, donuts, or potato chips. And not every stressor can be identified as easily as the examples given. Many people harbor resentment, anger, or fear deep within them from a situation or situations that occurred in their past. Their overeating behavior is a way they act out their repressed emotions, yet they may not realize it.

Your Relationship with Food

Consider the following questions:

- Do you often eat when you are frustrated or anxious?
- Does food help you feel calm and less nervous?
- Do you reach for food when you have to think about or confront a problem or challenge?
- Do you believe that people would accept you more or you would be more popular if you were thinner?
- Does food take the place of love or companionship when you are bored or lonely?
- Do you sometimes have episodes of binge eating when you feel you cannot control yourself?
- Do you ever induce vomiting or take excessive amounts of laxatives to eliminate food from your body?

If you answered "yes" to any of the above questions, you are not alone. Many overweight people use food as a drug because it offers them comfort and security or eases their pain. For some, it is the pain of low self-esteem; for others, it is the ache of not feeling loved or wanted. The stereotypical picture of a dejected woman sitting all alone with a pint of ice cream or a family-size bag of potato chips because she doesn't have a date that night is one with which many people can identify.

Psychiatrists also find that some people use food to shield themselves from the hurt associated with emotional, physical, or sexual abuse they suffered as children. Louis Aronne, M.D., author of *Weigh Less, Live Longer,* notes that weight problems are common among people who had a dysfunctional childhood. Naturally, not everyone who experienced family dysfunction during childhood overeats as an adult, but for many people the unconscious anxiety and painful memories can lead them to use food as a way to disguise or bury pain and hurt.

The use of food as a drug is a learned response. It is common, for example, for parents and other well-intentioned people to give sweets to children when they are upset or crying. Somehow, food is supposed to "make it all better," take away the hurt, pain, or confusion. Food can be a sign of love or a reward for good behavior: "finish your dinner and you'll get dessert"; "get good grades and I'll buy you ice cream." As an adult, you hold memories of those times in your subconscious and may turn to food when you need emotional healing or you need to feel good.

Regardless of the reason for which they were acquired, learned responses can be unlearned. The ideas and techniques discussed in Part Two of this book can help you take back control of your relationship with food. Once you understand that relationship, you can shed pounds and keep them off, permanently.

About 30 percent of people who seek help for serious weight problems are binge eaters. People who are binge eaters feel they cannot control how much they eat and so consume large amounts of food, often all at one time. Often they vomit the food or take excessive amounts of laxatives in an effort to avoid weight gain. This behavior is *bulimia* and can be life-threatening. Please see your physician if you are struggling with bulimia.

It's Not About Willpower

The intense desire to eat in response to emotionally over-whelming situations is biological. You may tell yourself that the next time you have a fight with your mother you won't console yourself with peanut butter and jelly sandwiches. But when the argument is over and you're in the middle of your third sandwich, you'll be blaming yourself for lack of willpower. The fact is, the stress has caused a reduction in the serotonin level in your brain. *Serotonin* is a hormone that naturally occurs in the brain. It is responsible for regulating mood, emotional well-being, and satiety. Communication between the mind and body is never-ending, and much of it occurs without our conscious knowledge. When you are under stress, your body responds in various ways: your heart rate may increase, your breathing may deepen, and adrena-line may enter your bloodstream. Your brain may also send signals to your body that cause different behaviors. When you are under prolonged periods of stress, it appears that the brain's stress-coping mechanism sends out a call for more serotonin. When it "sees" there isn't enough serotonin around, the brain knows the body needs to make more, and it needs the amino acid tryptophan to do it. So the brain sends out another signal that tells your body you need something sweet or starchy. Before you know it, you have your hand in the cookie jar or a giant bag of potato chips.

As the carbohydrates are digested, insulin is released into your bloodstream and amino acids are deployed. Among them is tryptophan, which is the slowest moving of all the amino acids. It eventually reaches your brain and the produc-tion of serotonin begins. Now your brain has what it needs, your stress level decreases, and you feel much less com-pelled to eat. You may, however, have finished off the bag of potato chips during the process.

Over about the next three hours, insulin levels decrease

and less and less tryptophan is available to the brain. Production of serotonin drops and may cease altogether. If you are still under stress, even if it is different stress, that craving for carbohydrates, for "comfort foods," will return.

The habit of eating in response to stress can be controlled in two ways. One is to follow an eating plan like that discussed in Chapter 3. Another is to learn how to manage your stress. These two approaches complement each other and when used together can improve your weight loss efforts and your overall well-being. In this chapter we explore the most powerful stress- and anxiety-reducing techniques—visualization/guided imagery, biofeedback, hypnotherapy, and meditation—that can complement your healthy eating and exercise program and help you get through stressful or rough times with a sense of calm and control. In each case, we offer you one or more sample exercises you can use the next time stress makes you want to reach for a chocolate bar.

Once you learn the techniques discussed in this chapter, you can use them again and again to help control stress, lose and maintain weight, ward off food cravings, and enhance your sense of well-being. They require only one special tool—your mind—and can be done whenever and wherever you are comfortable.

Visualization and Guided Imagery

Visualization is a general term used to describe the use of different visual techniques to achieve various physical, mental, emotional, and spiritual healing or other benefits. Guided imagery, which takes visualization several steps further, can be used to achieve the same goals. During visualization, people enter a relaxed state and focus their attention on a scene or image in their mind's eye. As the term implies, what you "experience" in your mind is primarily a visual image. In guided imagery, however, individuals take a mental "trip" through a scene they have chosen and call into play any perception associated with the senses: smell, feel, taste, sound, and sight. Both visualization and guided imagery are used for a wide variety of conditions and ailments, from obesity to arthritis and chronic pain. They are often used in conjunction with other natural healing methods, such as biofeedback, progressive relaxation, yoga, and tai chi. (See Biofeedback in this chapter; Yoga and Tai Chi in Chapter 9; and Appendix B.)

You can learn visualization and guided imagery on your own using tapes or self-help books, or you can study with someone who offers private or group sessions. Many people find tapes to be very helpful, especially in the beginning, to help them get started and discover what works for them. You can purchase prepared tapes for specific purposes, such as weight loss, stress reduction, and elimination of food cravings, or you can make your own tapes. This section contains a short guided-imagery script you can record and use to boost your metabolism, stimulate energy flow, reduce depression, and encourage you to exercise.

Visualization for Weight Loss

The following visualization is designed to boost your metabolism. It is only one of many different approaches you can use for weight loss. You may want to tape this imagery, or you can purchase guided-imagery tapes specially created for weight loss (see Appendix A for sources).

This visualization begins with deep breathing and leads you on a journey through your body. If you have never used guided imagery before, be patient. It may take you several sessions before you can create vivid scenes in your mind. To begin, choose a place where you won't be disturbed for about fifteen to twenty minutes. If you tape this session, pause five or more seconds at each ellipses (. . .).

Arrange your body so you are comfortable . . . allow your neck, head, shoulders, and spine to be straight and relaxed . . . Take a deep breath . . . as you breathe in, your mind becomes clearer and clearer . . . every time you breathe out, your mind becomes lighter. Continue to inhale slowly and deeply . . . fill your mind with light as you inhale . . . and release any tension as you exhale slowly and gently . . .

If any stray thoughts enter your mind, let them go as you exhale . . . send them out into the universe, riding on the back of any tension in your body . . . release those thoughts with each exhale . . . experience the stillness that remains . . . see the pure, shimmering light that remains in the stillness . . . Focus on the light as you take another deep breath . . . feel blessed by the stillness as you exhale . . .

Imagine you are in the center of the shimmering light . . . and as you float there in the stillness . . . sparkling light surrounds you . . . you feel the energy of the light as it moves all around you . . . around your feet . . . around your arms . . . around your legs . . . around your chest . . . around your head . . . it is touching every part of you with warm, loving tingles . . . feel the light enter your body . . . it is moving among your organs . . . it is dancing among your bones . . . it is flowing gently among your cells . . . it is moving up from your feet . . . all the way up your legs and into your pelvis . . . it is moving up through your chest . . . rising up through your throat and into your head . . . energizing every cell as it moves through your body . . . renewing every cell, every muscle, every part of you . . .

You sense that the light has a spirit, has an intelligence . . . as it moves through your body toward your energy source . . . it swirls around your pituitary gland at the base of the brain . . . it dances around the thyroid gland in your neck . . . and as it swirls and dances it gives them a command . . . it asks the glands to step up their production just a bit . . . to use just a little bit more energy . . . to let the engine run just a bit faster . . . filling you with more vitality . . .

Now notice that the body is responding . . . that all your cells are poised for the increase in energy . . . and the light moves among the cells, sending off sparks of energy . . . and you feel the increase in energy throughout your body . . . and your body feels lighter with the increase in energy . . . the muscles feel stronger . . . more fat cells shrink in size . . . your body feels strong at its new set point . . .

Feeling lighter and full of energy . . . you are still bathed with the light . . . completely invigorated by its power and what it has done for your body . . . knowing this lighter, alive body is yours . . . and knowing that you have done good work . . .

Feel yourself coming back . . . breathing gently and easily . . . let yourself and your new lighter body back whenever you are ready . . .

Hypnosis

Hypnosis is a natural state of mind in which you can take control of your body and mind using either the suggestions offered by a hypnotherapist or those you give yourself. This latter type of hypnotherapy, called *self-hypnosis,* is a skill that most people can develop with practice. It has proved to be successful for overweight people who are motivated to lose weight and who are willing to practice every day.

Before we explain how hypnosis can help you lose weight, let's clear up a few misconceptions about hypnotherapy.

• "I'll lose control of myself." Hypnosis is about having control, not losing it. When you are in a hypnotic trance, your level of awareness is altered, but you do not lose consciousness. In fact, the brain waves of people who are hypnotized show they are in a state of alert wakefulness.

• "I'm afraid I'll do something silly." While in a hypnotic trance, you will not do anything that goes against your ethics or principles. You maintain your free will at all times.

• "I can't be hypnotized." Have you ever been so engrossed in reading a book or watching a movie that you didn't realize an hour or more had passed? Have you ever been so focused on your own thoughts that you didn't hear someone talking to you or, if you were driving, remember how you got to your destination? You were in a hypnotic trance. Now imagine using your powers of focused concentration and suggestion for a specific purpose, such as curbing your appetite for sugar or stopping your desire to overeat. You can learn self-hypnosis, either with the help of a hypnotherapist or by using self-help books and tapes, to help you lose weight. Commercial lose-weight hypnosis seminars that attract large numbers of people generally are not effective. Save your money and time.

What Self-Hypnosis Can Do for You

Ninety-four percent of people who try hypnosis achieve some benefit, even if the only advantage is increased relaxation. In this section we focus on how you can use self-hypnosis to change your eating habits. You can customize the suggested sessions to match your specific needs. Do you want to eliminate your cravings for chocolate? Reduce your desire for potato chips and other fattening junk foods and increase your desire for fruits and vegetables? Direct yourself toward other activities when the desire to overeat hits you? You can use self-hypnosis for these and other desired goals. Once you learn self-hypnosis, you can practice it anytime you need it. It is much more useful and cost-effective than returning again and again to a hypnotherapist.

Losing Weight with Self-Hypnosis

People who overeat have their own particular reasons for doing so. Therefore you can choose techniques that are geared toward your special needs. According to Brian M. Alman, Ph.D., clinical psychologist and author of *Self-Hypnosis: The Complete Manual for Health and Self-Change,* there are several different methods to deal with overeating. You can use posthypnotic suggestions to do the following:

• Switch from one eating habit to another; for example, switch from snacking on high-calorie and high-fat foods, like chocolate, to munching on pretzels or hot air popcorn.

• Redefine your eating habits. First, select one or two of your poor eating habits, redefine them, and turn them into positive ones. For example: Now you eat a pint of ice cream three times a week. Accept the fact that you overeat, and redefine the amount to a half pint three times a week. After a while, redefine the amount to one cup, and so on until you are in control.

• Directly eliminate or significantly reduce undesirable habits. Here you can use posthypnotic suggestions aimed at self-control and at affirming that you are in control of your weight. For example: You always finish the food on your children's plates. You find yourself doing it without even thinking about it. You can use a posthypnotic suggestion to immediately scrape any leftovers into a container and save them for the dog or to put them into the trash or compost pile.

• Transform your desire to overeat into other activities. For example, the posthypnotic suggestion you choose can turn your trip to the refrigerator for ice cream into a walk around the block, time to curl up with a favorite book, or a telephone call to a friend.

Preparing for a Hypnotic Session

Regardless of the self-hypnosis techniques you use, the following guidelines can help you prepare for your sessions. These "generic" steps are followed by a self-hypnotic exercise. These sessions can help you eliminate stress and tension and a tendency to overeat. Relaxation is essential when changing eating habits, especially if you overeat in response to stress, anger, fear, or other strong emotions.

This exercise is only a sample; feel free to customize it to meet your unique needs and personality. Or you may want to write your own, use a commercial weight-loss hypnosis tape, or explore the suggestions in self-hypnosis books (see Appendix B for suggested readings). When choosing posthypnotic suggestions and cues for your sessions, remember these guidelines:

• Keep your suggestions positive. For example, say "I can visualize myself healthy and lighter," not "I see myself as overweight and undesirable." Prepare several positive suggestions.

• Prepare several posthypnotic cues, as some cues may be stronger for you than others.

Breathing Exercise

Andrew Weil, M.D., a leading authority on health and medical therapies and the author of *Natural Health, Natural Medicine,* recommends the following breathing exercise. It is an excellent way to start your day, a self-hypnosis session, a visualization session, and just if you're stuck in a line of traffic!

1. You can do this exercise in any position. However, if possible, keep your back straight as it facilitates breathing.
2. Place the tip of your tongue against the ridge behind and above your upper front teeth. Keep it there through the entire exercise.
3. Exhale completely through your mouth and make a "whoosh" sound as you do.
4. Inhale deeply and quietly through your nose to the count of 4. Keep your mouth closed.
5. Hold your breath for a count of 7.
6. Exhale through your mouth to a count of 8, making a "haaaaaaa" sound.
7. Repeat steps 4, 5, and 6 for a total of 4 breaths.

Self-Hypnosis for Stress Reduction and Overeating

• Choose a comfortable, quiet location where you will not be disturbed for about 30 minutes. During your first few sessions, you may need up to 15 minutes to fully enter a hypnotic state and focus on your goals. This is to be expected. Eventually, with practice, your entire session will be 10 minutes or less.

• Get into a comfortable position. Sit, lie down, relax in a recliner . . . it's up to you.

• Close your eyes or keep them open; again, the choice is yours. Many people close them once they enter the hypnotic state because it helps them focus more clearly.

• Deep breathing is an excellent way to begin your sessions, because it relaxes your entire body, clears your mind, and prepares you for easy passage into the hypnotic state. Refer to the deep breathing exercise above.

• Once you are comfortable and have begun deep breathing, focus your eyes on an object or spot that is in front of you and above your line of vision. It can be a clock on the wall, a tree outside your window, or a doorknob. Many people find that staring at a candle flame can be very hypnotic. Continue to concentrate on the item you have chosen and breathe slowly and deeply.

• Help yourself relax by repeating suggestions such as "As I breath in I inhale lightness. As I exhale I release all worries and tension." Your goal is to relax and free your mind of extraneous thoughts. You may also give yourself suggestions to close your eyes. "My eyelids feel heavy. As I close my eyes I experience a wonderful feeling of peace." Even after your eyes are closed, continue to reinforce the sense of peace and relaxation you feel. Here is where you can give yourself your first posthypnotic suggestion: "Whenever I want to rid myself of tension, I know that I can take several deep breaths and they will cause this relaxed, restful feeling I am feeling now."

Once you are in a hypnotic state, you can use the following self-hypnosis script, or your own variation of it, to reduce or eliminate stress and overeating.

Visualize a familiar object of your choice and concentrate on it in your mind. Repeat the following phrase over and over to yourself: "Nothing else exists except this _____." [I have chosen a daisy.] As you repeat "Nothing else exists except this daisy," imagine every detail of the flower—each petal, the stem, the leaves, the yellow center. Notice how the petals overlap; see the pollen on the yellow center. Continue to repeat the phrase until the words and the image totally consume your mind.

Now, one by one, see each petal separate from the yellow center and blow away. Watch each petal as it catches the wind and disappears, until each one is gone. Then let the leaves blow away, until all that is left is the stem. Now let the stem blow away and continue to concentrate on the spot where the daisy was but is no more. Stay in the middle of this quiet emptiness for several minutes and experience the relaxation.

As you allow yourself to savor the relaxed moment, give yourself the following suggestions and cues. "Many times during the day between meals, I get a craving for something sweet, like chocolate or cookies. Whenever this feeling comes over me, I open the refrigerator door if I'm at home; I open my desk drawer if I'm at work; I open my purse if I'm in my car or in public. Now when I get a craving, I will open up my notebook and write down my feelings. I will open my front door and take a brisk walk around the block. I will drink a glass of water. I will open up my eyes wider and see something in my environment that I had not noticed before. When I open myself up to these new possibilities, I will feel more in control. I will feel lighter and confident that I will achieve my weight goal."

Repeat these suggestions and cues several times.

Take a deep breath and push your stomach out. Hold it for several seconds and then breathe out and pull your stomach in as far as you can. Hold your stomach in for several seconds. Continue to practice this type of breathing four or five times. Each time you pull your stomach in, say to yourself "My stomach is getting smaller . . . now it will be easier for me to avoid sweets. I feel lighter and lighter with every breath I take."

Open your eyes and stretch your arms over your head. Take a deep breath and say to yourself: "Whenever I feel a craving for sweets, I have decided to open new doors. I will feel lighter and confident that I will achieve my weight goal."

Remember, you can customize your self-hypnotic sessions to address your specific eating habits and to follow your progress. Add to and change your posthypnotic suggestions and cues as needed. Below are some examples.

- "I can get more benefit and satisfaction from my food when I chew it slowly. I am full and satisfied and can stop eating before I finish everything on my plate when I chew my food slowly."
- "As I lose weight, I am proud of the way I look. I will find it easier and easier to keep the weight off. I am satisfied with how I am progressing."
- "I can enjoy trying new low-calorie foods, and I feel satisfied making them a part of my meals."

Biofeedback

People who are overweight and dieting are in constant communication with their body. It seems that there is no time people are more aware of hunger signals than when they are reducing the amount of food and calories they will consume! Biofeedback is a communication tool that opens the door to constructive dialogue between you and your body. It allows you to have more control over your eating habits and cravings, to improve your concentration, and to achieve an overall feeling of relaxation.

Biofeedback involves the use of a device (at least while you are learning the method) that measures what your body is doing *(bio-)* and lets you know what that response is *(feedback)* via some type of signal, such as a needle moving on a gauge or a series of beeps or blinking lights on a monitoring device. The monitors typically are electronic instruments that have electrodes that are placed on the skin over various muscles. The electrodes detect your body's physiological responses, such as skin temperature, muscle tension, blood pressure, and heart rate, and transmits them to the biofeedback machine, which then provides input on the responses.

You will need to work with a biofeedback therapist for at least several sessions until you learn how to "read" the signals passing between your mind and your body. Once you do, you will be able to practice biofeedback sessions without needing a monitor.

To demonstrate how biofeedback can help you relieve stress and reduce food cravings, we will look at how it worked for Kathleen, a thirty-two-year-old bookkeeper who wanted to lose 30 pounds. Kathleen was an admitted "junk food junkie" whose weaknesses included salty snacks such as potato chips and corn chips. She experienced a lot of stress on the job and kept stashes of her "comfort foods" in her desk. A friend had suggested biofeedback to her, but she was skeptical because she said she had "tried to relax" many times in the past without much success.

At the biofeedback clinic, the therapist explained that she would measure the amount of muscle tension at various sites on Kathleen's body. After she placed the sensors, the therapist asked Kathleen to think about her job for a few minutes. Then she asked her to concentrate on relaxing her muscles and releasing the tension from her body. The gauge on the machine indicated that Kathleen was not relaxing at all.

"But I'm trying to relax, I really am," she said. The therapist assured Kathleen that with the help of the monitor and visualization (see Visualization and Guided Imagery in this chapter), she would learn to relieve her stress and with it her overwhelming desire for her comfort foods. Visualization and biofeedback are a common and effective combination for the relief of stress and cravings.

Kathleen chose to concentrate on the most relaxing image she could think of: her parents' cabin in the mountains that she used to visit every summer as a teenager. She had vivid recollections of the smell of pine, the call of the owls late at night, and the cool water in the lake by the back door. After only six sessions over a three-week period, Kathleen was able to significantly decrease her stress level and began to reduce her cravings. With promises to practice the routine every day, she ended her sessions with the monitor and continued to use the biofeedback method at work or whenever her tension level sent her for the snack bags.

How Does Biofeedback Work?

The biofeedback equipment makes you aware of your body's own signals and abilities to control stress and the food cravings it creates. Your increased awareness of these signals can help you learn to make the mental and physical adjustments needed to relieve your stress and thus your desire to overeat. Biofeedback can be very effective for people who want to have greater control over their cravings and who commit themselves to practicing every day. The ongoing dialogue you establish between your mind and your body can be instrumental in helping you lose and maintain your desired weight.

Meditation

Bernie Siegel, M.D., who has done much research on meditation and its use in managing life-threatening and terminal illness, and who is the author of *Peace, Love, and Healing,* defines it as ''an active process of focusing the mind into a state of relaxed awareness.'' Regardless of the route people take to reach this state, Dr. Siegel notes that ''the result of all meditation methods is ultimately the same: to induce a restful trance which strengthens the mind by freeing it from its accustomed turmoil.''

There are two basic approaches to meditation: mindfulness and concentrative. Perhaps the best way to describe mindfulness is that it is like watching a parade: You focus your attention on passing thoughts, sensations, and feelings without becoming involved or concerned about them. You acknowledge their existence, but you do not become part of the street scene. Whenever you feel yourself drift into the thoughts, or into the parade, you gently bring your mind back to the sidewalk—back to concentration. This simple act of always bringing your mind back to focus is a form of mental exercise, says Joan Borysenko, Ph.D., author of *Minding the Body, Mending the Mind*. It flexes your "mental muscles of awareness and choice" and helps you better achieve the goals you have set for yourself.

When you practice concentrative meditation, you focus your attention on something repetitious: your breath, an image, a sound (such as a mantra), in order to calm your mind and increase your level of awareness. Concentrative meditation was proven to have significant scientific value back in the 1970s when Drs. Herbert Benson and R. Keith Wallace demonstrated that it decreased breathing rate, heart rate, and oxygen consumption after only a few weeks of practice.

Meditations for Weight Loss

Below are two short meditations. The first is a concentrative meditation in which you will concentrate not on your breath or a sound but on an action: the process of eating. You may want to start with just a snack, like an apple or some other small food item, the first few times. The second meditation is an example of mindfulness. Use it when you get a craving for a specific food or when you want to eat between meals.

There are commercial meditation tapes you can purchase and play every day to help you stay on course (see Appendix A). Some people find it helpful to tape meditations they find in books so they can just pop a cassette into their recorder and play the meditation of their choice.

Concentrative Meditation

This meditation is a bit different from what you usually expect, but keep an open mind. Try this meditation when you feel an urge to overeat or you are about to give in to a craving. Spend extra time doing deep breathing exercises if you need them. Then choose a simple food item—an apple or pear is a good choice.

1. Sit in a comfortable chair in front of a table and hold your spine straight. Place the food on the table and close your eyes.

2. Relax your shoulders, lift your chest, and let your chin fall lightly toward your throat.

3. Place your hands on your knees, palms up. Do some deep breathing exercises until you feel relaxed.

4. Once you feel calm, open your eyes slowly and look only at the piece of fruit before you. Slowly reach out with one hand and pick up the fruit. With your eyes on the fruit, raise the fruit to your mouth and take a bite. Return the fruit to the table and keep your eyes on it at all times.

5. Keep your eyes on the fruit on the table as you slowly chew the piece in your mouth. Focus completely on chewing the fruit. Notice how it feels in your mouth. Continue chewing it until it is liquid and then swallow it slowly. Notice how it feels going down your throat.

6. Wait a minute after you swallow the fruit and just let your eyes stay on the food in front of you. After one minute, slowly reach out with your hand and pick up the fruit again. Again, keep your eyes on the fruit as you raise it to your lips and take another bite. Return it to the table.

7. Continue this sequence until you have finished eating the fruit. Remember always to keep your eyes on the fruit. After you have finished chewing the last bite and you have swallowed it, sit quietly for a minute or two with your eyes closed and focus on your breathing.

Mindfulness Meditation

In this meditation you will explore your body and discover where you feel hunger. Once you find it, you will allow it to leave.

1. Find a spot where you can lie down and be comfortable for 20 to 30 minutes. Slowly stretch out and "check in" with your body parts as you stretch. Start with the soles of your feet, acknowledge how they feel, and then move upward, stopping at different body parts along the way until you reach the top of your head.

2. Allow your eyes to close; take a deep breath and slowly exhale.

3. As you inhale again, shift your breathing to your belly or a spot just below your navel. Allow your breath to come and go from that place, gently and slowly. Allow yourself to be fully aware of your breathing and the rise and fall of your abdomen.

4. After a moment, allow yourself to shift your focus and to become aware of your body. Ask yourself, Where do I feel hunger? Be a silent observer of your body. Allow your consciousness to move slowly and deliberately throughout your body. When you find a spot that harbors hunger, stop and explore it. What shape is the hunger? Is it long, tall, shallow, deep? Allow the hunger to assume a shape that has a bottom and sides. Let it be whatever it wants to be.

5. Once your hunger has created its shape, imagine the shape is filling up with water. Allow the space to fill with water, completely to the top.

6. Now visualize the water slowly leaving the space. Allow it to drain out of the space until it is completely gone. Once it is gone, allow the space to fill up again. If you have time, allow it to fill up and drain out a third time.

7. After you have allowed the water to drain out for the

last time, breathe in and be aware of any sensations in your body.

8. When you are ready to return, open your eyes and take a slow, deep breath. Release it slowly.

When you first begin this meditation, you will probably be very aware of the feeling of hunger. As the meditation continues, however, and you observe the water draining, the feeling of hunger will eventually decrease or disappear. Practice this meditation daily.

Reaping the Benefits

Daily meditation practice is important if you want lasting results. Ideally, you will establish a routine of, say, 15 minutes in the morning and another 15 or 20 minutes at night after work. Accumulate several meditations and switch them based on your mood and needs at the time. (See Appendix B for books that give examples of meditation techniques.)

Meditation has other benefits in addition to helping you control appetite and food cravings. For people with mild high blood pressure, meditation is often the recommended first line of therapy. Meditation also decreases the levels of stress hormones in the blood, reduces pulse and respiratory rate, boosts the immune system, induces the relaxation response, and increases the activity of alpha brain waves, which are the waves present during deep relaxation and creativity.

The ideas and exercises presented in this chapter can help you achieve mind over matter . . . food matters, as well as matters of stress. They open up a dialogue between your body and mind that, once established, can facilitate your healthy eating and exercise habits. Perhaps the best support you have to help you lose weight is your mind. Make friends with it, and keep it healthy, too.

CHAPTER NINE

Not Your Usual
Exercise Chapter

It's a well-known fact that aerobic exercise helps burn calories, and it is recommended for weight loss as well as for general overall fitness and health. However, *knowing* that something works and actually doing it are two different things. In this chapter we look at how you can add *fun and effective* aerobic exercise to your life. We also explore yoga and tai chi, two movement modalities that can stimulate your metabolism, increase flexibility, improve balance, promote overall well-being, improve muscle tone, and increase range of motion. Practicing either or both of these "exercises" can give you a sense of calm, self-esteem, confidence, and poise.

The "E" Word

According to the U.S. Public Health Service's *Healthy People 2000* (1991) report:

> Regular physical activity can help to prevent and manage coronary heart disease, hypertension, noninsulin-dependent diabetes mellitus, osteoporosis, obesity, and mental

health problems (e.g., depression, anxiety). Regular physical activity has also been associated with lower rates of colon cancer and stroke and may be linked to reduced back injury. On average, physically active people outlive those who are inactive. Regular physical activity can also help to maintain the functional independence of older adults and enhance the quality of life for people of all ages.

In terms of monetary and time investment, exercise is the best "buy" you can make for your health. The most popular form of aerobic exercise—walking—costs nothing except the price of a good pair of walking shoes. Jogging, swimming, biking, skiing, rowing, jumping rope, Stairmaster machines, dancing, aerobic classes, and other activities may require minimal outlay, more if you want to join a health club. And if you consider your choice of exercise to be entertainment as well, you're really getting a bargain!

Exercise CAN Be Fun

Exercise usually gets a bad rap, and one reason is that people keep thinking about it in a negative way. "I *have to* exercise," "Exercise is boring," "I don't have time to exercise," and "I'm too tired to exercise" are just a few of the consistently negative phrases associated with exercise. "The problem with exercise," said one overweight woman, "is that it has no taste, you can't sink your teeth into it, and it doesn't feel good. So why would I want to do it?" In this chapter, we want to change these negative words about exercise into positive ones. Perhaps we can't give exercise flavor, but we hope to make it less boring, and maybe even make it exciting. You'll see that you *do* have time to exercise, and that you'll feel much less tired once you do; in fact, you'll feel good! Let's see what you can "sink your teeth into"!

How Exercise Helps You Lose Weight . . . and More

When combined with a healthy eating plan, exercise helps you lose weight faster and helps you keep it off. This occurs because exercise increases your metabolic rate. A boost in metabolism means more calories burned. All it takes to raise your metabolic rate is 20 to 30 minutes of aerobic exercise. This increased metabolic rate can continue for 30 minutes or longer, depending on how strenuous your session is. The optimal number of aerobic sessions per week is four to five.

Exercise also changes your brain chemistry. After about 20 minutes of aerobic exercise, the brain increases its production of morphine-like substances called *beta endorphins,* the same compounds that create the "runner's high" many runners and other endurance athletes report. Twenty or more minutes of aerobic exercise, such as walking, can make you feel less depressed, less stressed, and emotionally lighter, healthier, and more positive. If you usually overeat because you are depressed or lonely, for example, a 30-minute brisk walk can put a positive spin on your mood, burn calories, and hopefully prevent you from overeating.

Exercise also has many other benefits. If you have diabetes, you already know that exercise is a critical part of maintaining proper blood sugar levels. It also strengthens the heart and circulatory system, boosts the immune system, increases muscle tone (which helps you burn more calories), relieves stress and depression, and improves flexibility and strength.

CAUTION: Before you begin any exercise program, consult with your physician. Together you can determine the best exercise program for you.

Words on Walking

We've mentioned many aerobic exercises you can try, yet perhaps the easiest and most versatile of them is walking.

Walking takes no special equipment or training, can be done just about anywhere, and can be incorporated easily into your daily routine. It is the exercise of choice of physicians and is especially suited for people who are overweight or who have heart problems or diabetes.

You've talked with your physician about exercising, so let's get moving! If you haven't exercised in a while, start your exercise program slowly. Begin with about 5 to 10 minutes of gentle stretching. Now you're ready to lace up your walking shoes and take off. Start slow and gradually increase your pace. You want to give yourself a good workout but not too much, so monitor your progress with the "walk and talk" test: if you can talk effortlessly while you are walking, you're not overexerting yourself. You can also check your heart rate to see if you have reached and are maintaining your target rate. Your *target heart rate* is the rate at which you burn calories effectively and condition your heart and muscles. See page 157 to determine what your target heart rate is. You want to exercise so that you maintain your target rate for 15 to 20 minutes, longer once you get in shape.

Variety = Fun
No one likes to be bored, and that's especially true when you are exercising. So instead of excuses for *not* exercising, we offer solutions to *combat* boredom.

• Team up with a friend or two and walk together. You may get so involved in talking that you walk longer and farther than you planned! Or you might join a walking club and make some new friends in the process. Some walking clubs meet and walk in indoor shopping malls, away from inclement weather and possibly undesirable street conditions.

• Have a sense of competition? Why not form a walk-across-your-state-or-the-country competition? There's nothing like the lure of competition and perhaps a prize at the end for the winner to get you up and moving. (See the box on page 157, Organizing a Walk-Across, for details.)

• Tune in to some music. Strap on the headphones and stroll with soul.

• Walking time gives you an excellent opportunity to listen to books on tape. Listening to an interesting book may even get you out walking more and longer, just so you can hear the rest of the story!

• Change your walking route whenever you can. If you like to walk in the morning before going to work, take your walk on the way to work instead of before you leave the house. Do you drive by a park or another nice area where you could stop and walk before continuing on to work? Just bring along your work shoes to change into once you're done. You could also walk during lunch or after work, or stop by a large indoor shopping mall and walk in air-conditioned comfort and safety.

• If possible, break up your walking routine by using a treadmill, stair-climbing machine, or ski machine. Or, if you prefer, use a stationary bike or go swimming. It is important to vary your exercise, not only to avoid boredom but also to work and strengthen other muscles.

Variety Adds More Than Spice

Many weight loss experts recommend that you change your exercise routine occasionally, or even frequently, to break the pattern your body becomes accustomed to. This break in routine often kick-starts a stalled weight-loss program and may increase the amount of weight you lose. It is uncertain whether this effect is psychological or physiological, but any change generally causes the body to respond.

You don't need a lot of money or equipment to add variety

to your exercise sessions. Help can be as close as your local library. Check out their video section for aerobic, tai chi, and yoga tapes (see Tai Chi and Yoga in this chapter) you can try in the privacy of your living room. Invite a friend over to join you and hold your own "mini aerobics class." If you would like to use a stationary bike and don't have one, ask your friends and relatives. Many people have a stationary bike stowed away in their house, idle and just waiting for someone like you to use it.

Swimming is an excellent aerobic activity for people who are overweight and who may have problems with weight-bearing exercise. Inaccessibility to a pool and the high cost of many health clubs can be a barrier. However, if you can occasionally get to a pool and use swimming as an alternative to walking, it will be very beneficial. Even if you don't know how to swim, walking in waist-high water provides an excellent workout. Also see if your local Y or community recreation facilities offer water aerobics classes. These are often inexpensive and fun.

Intensity Is Key

You have to heat it up to lose it, according to researchers reporting in *Behavioral Medicine* (vol. 2, no. 1 [Spring, 1995]:31–39). A leisurely stroll around the park is probably not going to raise your body temperature enough to be effective in weight loss. Recent scientific research shows that unless you move enough to increase your body temperature, don't expect any weight loss to come of your efforts. Some researchers say swimming is not an effective weight loss exercise because water takes heat away from the body; however, not all experts agree on this point. Brisk walking is still the exercise of choice among physicians and researchers.

Organizing a Walk-Across

You need a group of walkers—the more the merrier—but as few as four will do. Determine the distance you want to walk and your destination, starting in your city. If this is the first time you've planned such an event, keep the goal reasonable so the participants don't lose enthusiasm or feel discouraged. For example, say you live in Chicago. Choose a point across the county within a 100- to 150-mile radius. Create a simple map of the route from Chicago to your chosen destination. If possible, display the map on a board or wall so you can plot the progress of each walker. Choose a starting date and then, as each person takes a walk during the coming week, he or she reports the number of miles walked. The number of miles is recorded on a running tally for each person. To make it more visual and exciting, you can use pushpins with people's names on them and move the pins along the route on the map. The first person to "walk" to the other city wins a little prize—something not related to food, of course. This simple event builds self-esteem and a sense of accomplishment, and helps burn calories. After the success of your first Walk-Across, you can plan longer ones, perhaps across the state or even the country!

Determine Your Target Heart Rate

- Subtract your age from the number 220 (for example, if you are 40 years old, 40 from 220 is 180).
- To determine the heartbeat range you want to achieve during exercise, take 60 percent of 180 ($0.60 \times 180 = 110$) and 85 percent of 180 ($0.85 \times 180 = 153$).
- A healthy heart rate for you to achieve during exercise is

110 to 153 beats per minute. If you are new to exercising, you want to stay at the low end of the range.

- To check your heart rate while exercising, place the tip of a finger on your pulse on the thumb side of your wrist or on the side of your neck. Count the beats for 10 seconds and then multiply that number by six.

Tai Chi

Tai chi chuan (tai chi) is an integrated exercise system that originated in ancient China in about 3000 B.C. The literal translation of *tai* is "great" and *chi* is "ultimate energy." The art of tai chi involves the generation and feeling of energy through movement. It has been called slow-motion calisthenics, moving meditation, or poetry in motion. It brings together the Chinese philosophy of yang (positive) and yin (negative), the eternal opposites. As people practice tai chi, they move from yin to yang (soft, slow, rest; to hard, fast, motion) and vice versa in a flowing, harmonious balance.

But don't let tai chi's slow motion fool you. Its inherent slowness is the source of its strength. The Chinese explain that as you develop greater slowness, you increase your ability for greater speed, flexibility, endurance, and strength. Tai chi can stimulate proper function of the internal organs and circulation of blood and lymph.

Tai Chi for Weight Loss
Tai chi has several features that make it an ideal form of physical activity for people who are overweight. Tai chi:

- is composed of gentle, nonstrenuous movements. Because it is not physically demanding and you can progress at your own pace, perform only those motions that are comfortable for you.

- promotes relaxation and helps build coordination and strength, all of which contribute to overall well-being.
- involves graceful, flowing motions that have been described as "poetry in motion." Some overweight people feel uncomfortable and encumbered by their excess weight. Tai chi allows them to feel light and balanced; they report feeling better about themselves.
- stimulates the proper function of many systems throughout the body, including the thyroid gland, which is responsible for metabolism.

Tai chi is a holistic blend of physical movement, breathing exercises, and meditation. Meditation is a vital component of tai chi, and together with the physical movements it relieves stress and boosts the immune system.

You can learn tai chi from the few well-illustrated books on the market (see Appendix B). However, the recommended way to learn tai chi is to take a course so you can have professional help while acquiring the basics. Then you may want to follow up with a book or video. Many community centers, hospitals, and schools either sponsor or offer tai chi classes, for beginners to advanced students. Classes usually last six to eight weeks, after which you can move to the next level if you wish.

When choosing a tai chi instructor, ask about the philosophy of the class. Many instructors focus on the physical health benefits and the calm, relaxed nature of the art, while a few focus on the martial arts aspects. Naturally, those who emphasize the latter need to be avoided at this stage. Before beginning tai chi, consult with your doctor.

Traditional tai chi includes more than one hundred movements. Over time, many modified forms have been created, and today most practitioners use 24 to 48 positions. Below are just a few of those positions to get you started.

MOVEMENT 1: STRIKE PALM TO ASK BUDDHA
(SEE FIGURE 9–1)

- Stand straight, feet together and hands to your sides.
- Turn your right foot outward 45 degrees.
- Bend both knees and extend your left foot forward about two feet. Keep the left knee straight, your heel on the ground, and your toes up.
- Raise both arms to shoulder level and face palms forward.
- While keeping your arms up, bring your hands together until they almost touch. Your hands should be about 18 inches from your chest.
- Keeping your hands open, bend the right hand at the wrist so it is now perpendicular to the middle of the left hand. Hold this position for several seconds.

MOVEMENT 2: GRASP BIRD'S TAIL (SEE FIGURE 9–2)

- From the ending position of movement 1, move your left foot back past your right heel until it is 45 degrees in back of your right foot. Your left foot should be perpendicular to your right foot and the right toes should point up.
- Move your hands down to waist level and diagonal to your left hip. Keep both elbows bent slightly, your left palm up and the right palm down. Your right leg should be straight and the toes up.
- Bring your right leg back until the ball of the right foot touches the arch of the left foot.
- Step forward and diagonally with your right foot. Bend both knees and center your weight. Keep your back straight.
- Twist at the waist and shoulder until your hands are even.

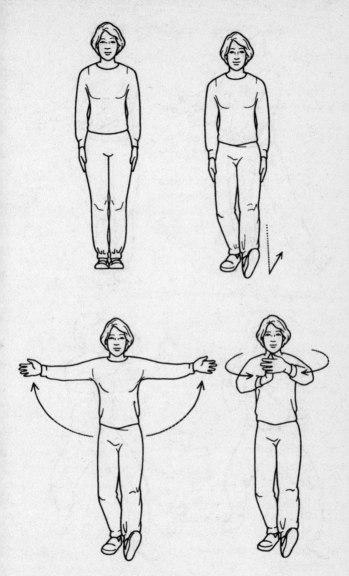

Figure 9–1.

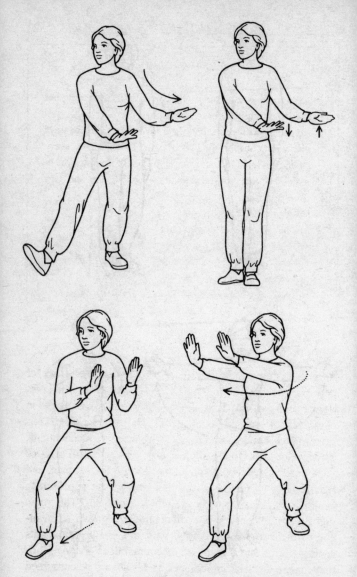

Figure 9–2.

Tai Chi Practice Tips

- Keep moving at all times. Tai chi is not about posing but about keeping the chi in motion.
- Be patient with yourself. Tai chi involves moving in ways that you probably are not used to; for example, every movement must include your entire body. It takes time to remember that you need to move your arms and legs simultaneously.
- Practice every day.
- Matching your movement with your breathing may seem difficult at first, but it will come easily with practice. Your movements should be even and flowing and in harmony with your breathing.
- Visualize tension and fat melting away as you move.

Yoga

Yoga has come a long way from its stereotypical image of people in turbans sitting cross-legged on the floor. The practice of yoga has spread around the world and can be found in communities big and small across the United States. It is practiced by children and the elderly; teachers, accountants, students, doctors, police officers, and store clerks all practice yoga to relax, lose weight, maintain health, reduce pain, and reduce fatigue. Yoga is a way of living whose approach to health is the balance of body, mind, and spirit. The yogic diet promotes consumption of organically grown (if available) fruits, vegetables, grains, nuts, and seeds. Stimulants such as coffee and alcohol are discouraged, as are any foods that contain artificial ingredients. Meals should be consumed in a nonstressful environment without distractions. This dietary approach promotes efficient digestion. As you can see, a yogic dietary approach is very similar to the healthy eating habits discussed in Chapter 3.

There are several types of yoga, most of which focus on spiritual awareness and enlightenment. Hatha yoga, however, is a mind-body approach that combines physical healing with meditation. In hatha yoga, you stretch, strengthen, and heal your body using fluid, gentle movements while you focus your mind on your breathing and physical sensations. Your mind and body work as one to heal.

Getting Started with Yoga

Before you begin a yoga program, discuss your plans with your physician or other health care provider to assess your general health and flexibility. If you have back problems or if you are pregnant, there are some positions you should avoid. You and your health care professional can choose the yoga positions that are best for you.

There are many excellent books and videos available to help you learn different yoga positions. We recommend, however, that you first attend at least a few sessions with a yoga instructor, either individually or with a group, so you can learn proper breathing technique and receive any help you may need in getting started with a yoga program. Try to find an instructor who has experience in working with overweight people. (See the Appendixes for books and videos and how to find an instructor.)

Yoga and Weight Loss

Yoga can help you control craving and overeating in two ways. One, yoga is a discipline that gives you mastery over your mind while it relaxes you. When you remove the feeling of urgency that is associated with stress and food cravings, you build up self-control and inner mastery. Two, it is a gentle form of exercise that promotes circulation and metabolism and a sense of well-being.

Below are four yoga poses (or *asanas*) recommended for obesity. There are many others; see Appendix A for more information, or ask your yoga instructor. These asanas are designed to gently stimulate circulation, stretch tight muscles, strengthen weak ones, and improve posture. Do them slowly and do not push yourself. Practice these and other beginning poses daily for a month or more before you attempt more advanced poses. Read the box below before you get started. If possible, have a friend join in the fun!

Yoga Prep and Tips

- Practice yoga in front of a mirror if possible so you can see how you move.
- Wear comfortable clothing that allows you to see your body in motion. Suggestions: shorts and a T-shirt, leotards, or a swimsuit; no sweatpants
- Bare feet are a must.
- The following accessories are useful for some poses:
  —a folded or rolled-up hand towel for under your neck; a bath towel for under your head
  —a folded bath towel for under your lumbar area
  —a nonskid mat if you are not practicing on a nonskid floor. Proper alignment of your head, neck, and back are important, so experiment with the placement and thickness of the rolls and pads until you are comfortable.
- Proper breathing is vitally important when practicing yoga. Some things to remember:
  —inhale and exhale through your nose
  —as you inhale, relax the muscles in your face, neck, and shoulders and focus on maintaining correct posture
  —as you exhale, perform the movement of the pose
  —never hold your breath
  —when you focus on your breathing during yoga, you

> derive the benefits of stress reduction and increased self-awareness.
>
> • If possible, practice yoga 15 to 30 minutes a day at least five days a week. If you have only five minutes to spend one day, five minutes is better than nothing.

Pose 1: Tree Breathing

Stand upright with your feet comfortably apart and your arms down in front of you and your fingers interlocked. Your palms should be facing down. Take a deep breath, and as you inhale, rise up on your toes. As you rise up, raise your hands up to chest level and then up over your head. Reach upward and feel the stretch from your ankles to your fingers. Then, as you exhale, lower your arms and come down on your heels. Repeat this sequence five more times.

Pose 2: Forward-Backward Bending

Stand with your feet comfortably apart and arms at your sides. As you inhale, stretch your arms up over your head and lean backward slightly, bending your spine. Go only as far back as is comfortable. As you exhale, straighten up and then bend forward as far as you can with your arms still extended. Repeat this backward and forward motion, inhaling and exhaling with the corresponding movement, five or six more times. Gradually increase the speed at which you bend back and forth, but only what is comfortable.

Pose 3: Embryo

Lie on the floor with your heels together and your arms stretched out behind you. Breathe normally throughout this pose. Inhale slowly and as you do, bend your knees and raise your legs. Then, as you exhale, bring your knees in toward your chest. Hold your knees with interlocked fingers and lift your chin toward your knees as close as you can. Next, extend your left leg at a 45-degree angle to the floor and rotate it slowly, five times in a clockwise direction and five times in a counterclockwise direction. Bring your left leg back toward your chest, clasp it with interlocked fingers, and repeat the rotating sequence with your right leg. When you are done, hug both knees to your chest and rock back and forth on your back a few times.

Pose 4: Inverted Corpse

Lie near a wall and raise your legs so they are resting on the wall, either at a 45-degree angle or vertically. Do not bend your knees. Relax. Practice this pose after doing a series of active poses, especially those you do lying down, like the Embryo above.

The Inverted Corpse pose is an ideal position to use when you are experiencing food cravings or a desire to overeat. Once you are in position, close your eyes and repeat to yourself: "I want to eat, and I will allow myself to do so, but first I want to calm my mind and my body. I want to enjoy the food and know that it is nourishing my body because I deserve to be nurtured." Then take five slow, deep breaths and repeat the following: "Now when I eat I will eat slowly and savor each bite."

Now be honest: didn't you have some fun? And the fun can continue, day after day, especially as you see and feel the results of your efforts. In addition to looking better, exercise can give you more energy and help you feel more confident and poised. Thus, your loss is also your gain!

CHAPTER TEN

How to Make Natural Weight Loss Work for You

You've turned over the last page of Chapter 9 and you're excited. Many of the holistic methods you've read about sound intriguing, so you've decided to try the natural approach to weight loss. However, you don't know anyone who has tried dandelion tea or reflexology or spirulina or tai chi. And there are so many choices, and some of them are so tempting . . .

Using What You've Learned

This book has introduced you to an array of safe, natural weight-loss options. It is now up to you to take the steps to a healthier, lighter you.

• Reread the chapters on nutrition and exercise. Any successful weight loss and maintenance plan must include these two components.

• Go back through the book and choose two or three of the techniques and supportive remedies that appeal most to you. One of your choices should include some type of stress reduction plan.

• Write down your plan of action and post it where you can see it. Put one on your refrigerator, on your bathroom mirror, on the visor in your car, in the top drawer of your desk . . . anywhere it can remind you and reinforce your choices.

To help you see how these steps can work for you, we present three different women who share their stories of how they lost weight using approaches discussed in this book. Their stories could be yours, yet no two situations are alike. Every individual comes to the weight loss arena with a unique set of inherited characteristics, emotional needs, medical conditions, and lifestyle habits. The secret to permanent weight loss is no secret at all: a commitment to make healthy changes in your life, a willingness to listen to your body, and a positive attitude.

Nowhere in this book do we tell you to count every calorie you eat. That's because when you listen to your body and treat it with respect by feeding it nutritious food; when you take control of the stress in your life rather than let it control you and your eating habits; when you choose supplements and herbs that support your weight loss efforts; when you take the time to be in your body and appreciate it for its health and vitality, even if you do not meet society's unrealistic body-type standards, you don't need to count calories unless you have a specific medical reason to do so. You do, however, need to be aware of the factors that can contribute to your being overweight so you will be better armed to deal with them.

That is precisely what Angela, Donna, and Stella did when they decided to lose weight naturally. First, Angela's story.

Angela

Angela is 29 years old and has two children ages 2 (Shawna) and 4 years (Jason). She is five feet four inches tall and at the time she started her natural weight-loss program, she weighed 170 pounds. Her body mass index (BMI) was 29; women with a BMI of 27.3 or greater are considered obese.

Throughout high school and college, Angela had fluctuated from 120 to 130 pounds but then added the rest of the weight after the birth of her children. While she was pregnant with Jason, Angela gained 35 pounds and kept 25 of it after the birth. She stayed at 150 to 155 until she was pregnant with Shawna, when she gained another 30 pounds. Before she became pregnant with Shawna, Angela had taken diet pills ("they made me feel speedy and nauseous"), joined a health spa for several months and tried the aerobics classes ("I felt fat and ugly next to some of those skinny women"), cut her caloric intake to 800 calories a day ("I was tired, dizzy, cranky, and *starving*"), and enrolled for a short time in a commercial weight-loss program. ("The more I lose the more I pay . . . now *that's* some incentive, isn't it?")

Each venture into a weight loss plan resulted in some weight loss—as much as 10 pounds at one point—but she gained it all back plus more. After Shawna was born, she returned to work part-time as a CPA. She tried several "$39.95 television weight-loss snake-oil specials," as she called them, and was contemplating phen-fen just before it was removed from the market and the decision was made for her. That's when she read about natural weight-loss methods and decided to give them a try. She set a 40-pound weight loss as her goal, got a notebook, and recorded everything she ate and drank for one week.

Angela's "Old" Lifestyle Plan

As Angela reviewed her diary at the end of the week, she made some interesting observations. Angela consumed four to six cans of soda a day, beginning early in the morning. Not all the sodas contained caffeine, so the attraction did not appear to be the caffeine. Her eating habits were poor. She started each day with a soda while she got the kids ready to take to her mother's and she got dressed for work. "Breakfast" consisted of finishing whatever the kids didn't eat on their plates, which typically was a sugary cereal or frozen waffles with syrup. She drank another can of soda on the way to work and then had one or two more during the morning to get her through to two o'clock, when she left to pick up her children at her mother's house. "Lunch" this particular week was defined as half a bagel with cream cheese, consumed at her desk at around one o'clock; "two bites" of pizza offered by an office co-worker; and "a piece or two" of donuts that are part of the office coffee station. On weekends she did not prepare lunch for herself but did "clean up" her kids' plates, which included part of a bologna sandwich on one day and chicken noodle soup on another.

After she brought the kids home in the afternoon, Angela always prepared a snack of peanut butter and jelly or cheese and crackers for the kids and would take just "a nibble or two" herself as she downed another soda. Dinner was served between six-thirty and seven P.M. and usually centered around ground meat, pasta, fried chicken, or hot dogs. Vegetables and fruits were glaringly absent. Angela ate a moderate amount for dinner, accompanied by yet another soda, and always had a late-night snack of ice cream, cookies, or some other sweets. There was no scheduled exercise in her diary, although she did write down that she had walked around the mall for 30 minutes one day while Shawna was taking her ballet lesson. That walk was interrupted, however, when Angela stopped to have a nonfat yogurt cone.

Angela often felt tired, and before her period she had an intense craving for chocolate and experienced lots of bloating. She moved her bowels only every two days, and at times she had to take a laxative for constipation. She often experienced gas pains shortly after dinner or whenever she actually ate breakfast or lunch.

Angela's New Lifestyle Plan

Angela developed the following plan for herself:

• Because she felt she could not get through her day without her ''soda fix,'' Angela believed she had a sugar addiction. She used the sugar withdrawal program, which includes vitamin C, chromium, and glutamine (see Chapter 4) for about four weeks.

• To replace the sodas, Angela drank naturally flavored seltzer water.

• At the same time, she established a balanced eating plan that included three healthy meals a day and eliminated the empty calories (sodas, ''bits and pieces'' she picked on during the day). Angela's first step was to stock up on items that are nutritious and easy to prepare and that her kids would eat, too.

Because Angela was always rushed in the morning, she bought instant oatmeal and cream of wheat, whole-grain bagels (she kept a supply in the freezer), frozen hash browns (without fat), raisins, rice cakes, and all-fruit jellies. She brought rice cakes, whole-grain crackers, and fresh fruit with her to work for lunch or a snack. Because Angela's work schedule did not allow her a standard lunch time, Angela opted to have a late-morning snack and then another snack when she picked up her kids in the afternoon. To fit in some exercise time, Angela asked her mother to watch the kids a bit longer three days a week so she could take a brisk thirty-minute walk around the park near her office.

• Angela gradually introduced vegetables and more beans and grains into her menus. To help promote bowel function so she would have at least one bowel movement a day, she took one teaspoon of psyllium seeds twice a day dissolved in water until her dietary fiber had increased to at least 30 mg a day.

• To facilitate the movement of fiber through her system, Angela made a point to drink at least eight glasses of water a day. To help her get sufficient water as well as to eliminate the gas pains she was experiencing, Angela drank an 8-ounce glass of water with the juice of a freshly squeezed lemon in it 30 minutes before each meal.

• Three weeks after starting her new program, Angela started a yoga class once a week. She found that she enjoyed it so much she practiced yoga nearly every day for at least 10 or 15 minutes.

• A natural complement to yoga is meditation, and Angela found that daily meditation not only was a good prelude to yoga, it also helped her reduce her sugar and chocolate cravings.

• To help reduce water weight and bloating before her menstrual period, Angela got relief from juniper berry tea taken for three to four days before her period.

Angela Eight Months–Plus Later

At eight months, Angela was just 5 pounds shy of her goal of 40. Six months later, she is still holding at 135 and her BMI is 23. She says she feels like a new person and has finally signed up for the aerobics class she once had to leave because she felt "too fat" to stay. Angela is not the only one who has benefited from her healthy eating habits: she has gradually replaced the kids' bologna and sweetened breakfast cereals with bean burritos and oatmeal and thrown away the white sugar and substituted dried fruit and honey.

Donna

Donna is a 43-year-old mother of two teenagers: 16-year-old Justin and 17-year-old Carl. She has been divorced for six years and works full-time as a marketing manager. At five feet six, she has weighed about 174 pounds since she was 20. Her BMI was 28. Both her parents were obese, as is her older sister, Fay. Donna had made several attempts to lose weight since her divorce, including use of over-the-counter diet pills, numerous attempts to fast, and a yearlong association with Weight Watchers, during which she lost 20 pounds but gained 27 once she left the program. Two things convinced Donna to try to lose weight again: the death of her mother from heart failure and diabetes; and Fay's recent diagnosis of noninsulin-dependent diabetes. As Donna said: "I don't like the direction my life could be going if I don't do something about it now." She also had another incentive: she had set her sights on an eligible bachelor who had just moved into her apartment complex.

Donna contacted an orthomolecular M.D. recommended to her by a co-worker who was trying to lose weight too. She prepared her food and exercise diary and brought it with her on her visit to Dr. S. After Donna completed her personal and family medical histories, Dr. S conducted a physical examination and explained the diagnostic tests he would perform in order to rule out any infections or any problems with her thyroid or digestive tract. His nurse then drew a blood sample as he explained that it would help him determine her enzyme, nutrient, and hormone levels and how they were working together. After noting that Donna had a family history of diabetes and that she had never been tested for diabetes, he scheduled a fasting glucose tolerance test for her. Donna told Dr. S that she had been feeling very tired for many months but had attributed it to working too hard and being overweight.

Donna's "Old" Lifestyle

Donna's diary revealed a woman who ate out a great deal, worked long hours, and had no scheduled time for exercise. Breakfast was usually juice and coffee while she got ready for work and then another cup of coffee while she drove to work. Several times a week she had breakfast meetings, and on those days she had Danish or a bagel and coffee. Lunch often meant having a Reuben sandwich with a client or sharing pizza or burgers with co-workers. Dinner was either takeout from a nearby Chinese restaurant, burgers from a fast-food restaurant, or a frozen dinner and a glass of wine. Often she had to work late either at the office or at home and it wasn't unusual for her to consume the greater portion of a 12- or 16-ounce box of cheese or wheat crackers while she worked.

Donna's Diagnosis and Plan

Donna's diabetes test came back positive. Given her mother's death and her sister's similar diagnosis, Donna felt a great deal of stress around her health. Dr. S assured her they could work together to control her diabetes, bring her weight down, control her food cravings, and relieve the stress she was feeling, all without the need for any type of medication. The doctor especially wanted to avoid using any oral diabetic drugs, as they are associated with weight gain (see Chapter 1).

The first consideration was to change Donna's diet. Dr. S recommended a modified version of Dr. McDougall's plan for diabetes and weight loss (see *McDougall's Medicine* in Appendix B for the full program), which calls for 80 to 90 percent carbohydrates, 5 to 12 percent protein, 5 to 10 percent fat, high fiber, and no cholesterol. Donna's plan would include 70 percent carbohydrates and 15 percent each protein and fat. Overweight individuals who follow McDougall's plan typically lose six to fifteen pounds of fat per month without feeling hungry and while keeping their blood sugar levels in balance. The plan is designed so people can follow it for a lifetime. Dr. S decided to use a modified version of the plan because he believed the full program was too big of a change for Donna.

Basically, Donna's meals were to revolve around starchy (for example, corn, potatoes) and all other vegetables, whole grains, pastas, beans, legumes, fruits, and soy products. She was encouraged to use salt-free and low-sodium seasonings and to substitute herbs when possible. Instead of sugar she could use honey, pure maple syrup, or no-sugar pure fruit spreads in small amounts.

With Dr. S's help, Donna developed menu ideas that fit into her busy schedule. Breakfast typically included fresh fruit plus a whole-grain hot cereal or whole-grain bagel with no-sugar jelly. Because Donna eats out a lot, she needed to take special care when ordering in restaurants. She soon learned that it was quite easy: if she ordered from the appetizer section (baked potatoes with salsa on the side, sides of steamed vegetables, brown rice, black beans) and if she asked for her pasta plain with sauce on the side or her vegetables steamed with herbs, the restaurants were glad to accommodate her. Dinners consisted of pasta primavera, stir-fry tofu and vegetables, and hearty stews and soups Donna learned to make in her new slow-cooker.

Donna was concerned about her cravings for crackers and other carbohydrates. A co-worker suggested she try self-hypnosis to help her get over the urges. After one session with a hypnotherapist and borrowing a book and tape on the subject from a friend, she began to practice self-hypnosis every day. Job stress was one of the reasons she felt she had these cravings, so some stress management was recommended by Dr. S. Exercise was at the top of the list, especially because of the diabetes and because Donna had not been getting any daily exercise. In addition to a walking program—30 minutes of brisk walking at least three times a week—he recommended she explore meditation and yoga, two complementary disciplines that could calm her mind as well as move and strengthen her body. He also prescribed 1,000 mg of evening primrose oil because of the history of obesity in her family, and 30 mg of Co-Q-10 three times a day, also for the obesity.

Donna's "New" Lifestyle

After three months Donna had lost 14 pounds: not as many as she had wished, but she was feeling much more energetic. Her digestion problems had cleared up, but she was experiencing some bloating associated with PMS. For this she started drinking dandelion tea, two cups twice a day the week before her menstrual cycle, and found some relief.

After six months she had lost an additional 10 pounds and was still practicing her yoga, although her self-hypnosis sessions had decreased significantly. With some encouragement from the friend who had recommended she try the hypnosis, she started to practice it regularly again and added suggestions to help her stay on her healthy eating plan. At one year, Donna had lost a total of 38 pounds and felt wonderful. Her diabetes was under control. She got some added incentive to continue her weight loss efforts by sharing recipes and menu ideas with her sister Fay, and the two sometimes take walks together for exercise.

Stella

At 26, Stella is five feet, one inch and weighed 126 pounds. Over the past six years she had "lost the same 10 to 15 pounds" three or four times using various meal replacement plans and diet pills. Stella was a postgraduate student in chemistry, and her goal was to lose 15 pounds—and keep it off—for her graduation in seven months.

Stella's "Old" Lifestyle

Stella kept a food and activity diary for one week. She always took time for breakfast: usually cold cereal with fruit and a cup of tea. It was a 30-minute bus ride to the university, where she put in long hours in the lab and tutoring. Lunch was a hurried affair that she consumed at her desk or in between students: fruit and some crackers, cookies, or granola bars. During the afternoon she usually drank two diet sodas. Two nights a week she stayed at school until eight to help with a special project, and on those nights she didn't eat dinner until she arrived home around nine. On the other three nights she arrived home at seven. She typically prepared herself some soup or a frozen dinner entrée, which satisfied her for about an hour before she gave in to her cravings for salty snacks—pretzels, potato chips, and cheese snacks. On weekends Stella spent time with her boyfriend and their friends, often eating out and drinking and snacking late into the evening.

Stella's "New" Lifestyle

Here's what Stella's new lifestyle plan looked like:

• Food: To avoid feeling so hungry at night, Stella adjusted her midday eating to include a hearty soup (vegetable, lentil, split pea, barley) or a salad with $\frac{1}{2}$ cup rice or beans and some fruit. She eliminated the diet sodas and replaced them with naturally flavored seltzer waters. On nights she arrived home late, she ate steamed vegetables with salsa or a small amount of grated low-fat cheese and whole-grain crackers. On the remaining nights she had pasta with marinara sauce and a green salad, a bean burrito with no-fat beans, stir-fry vegetables and tofu or 1 ounce of chicken, or some of the other healthy recipes she was finding in her recipe search.

• Supplements: Stella added 250 mg of chromium

picolinate after breakfast and 500 mg of garcinia cambogia after breakfast, lunch, and dinner to stimulate her metabolism. She also had a cup of sea wrack tea after dinner, which, along with the chromium, helped her curb her cravings for snack foods.

• Exercise: Stella got up 30 minutes earlier each morning so she could get off the bus a mile from her usual stop and walk to work. She admitted she was successful "80 percent of the time." She also decided to take advantage of the fitness facilities at the university, which were free because she was a postgrad student and an employee. Stella added 30 minutes of swimming to her weekend schedule and talked her boyfriend into joining her.

• Reflexology: Stella knew from past experience that her cravings for snack foods had gotten her "into trouble." Though she was taking the chromium and sea wrack, she wanted "triple protection" and learned the reflex points for appetite suppression and food cravings.

Stella Seven Months Later and Beyond
One month before her graduation, Stella reached her goal of 111 pounds. She walked up to receive her diploma one month later at 109, and she has hovered between 109 and 112 for more than six months.

Your Story

Here's where your story can begin. Resolve to take the first step. Explore new natural ways to control your weight. If possible, find a friend to share your new experiences with you. Your story will be different from that of any other person who wants to lose weight. And it can be a story that inspires another person to write his or her own story too.

CHAPTER ELEVEN

Where to Turn for Help

It's comforting to know there are knowledgeable, professional people you can turn to for help or encouragement as you embark on and continue with your weight loss program. In this chapter we offer you suggestions on how to choose the professionals who can assist you with your weight loss strategies. We explain what you can expect if you choose to visit a physician or various holistic health providers. Losing weight and keeping it off is a challenge, and we encourage you to seek assistance from health care professionals as well as support from family and friends. Make it a team effort!

If you decide to make such a visit, you may become more aware of all the factors that can affect your ability to lose weight and maintain your desired weight. This knowledge will let you know which strategies will best achieve your goal. Thus armed with the facts and natural approaches to help you along, you can begin your journey to a lighter, healthier you.

Contacting a Physician

As you've seen in Chapter 1, there are many factors that can contribute to being overweight, and so you may want to seek advice and assistance from professionals in different disciplines. If you need help in locating any of the categories of health care providers below, please see Appendix A for a listing of professional organizations that offer referrals and information, or check the listings in the Yellow Pages of your local telephone directory under each individual specialty, such as hypnotherapy or acupuncture. Also, ask your friends, family, and co-workers for referrals.

For help with the mainstay of any weight loss program, you will need help with eating habits and exercise. Be a discriminant shopper when looking for a medical professional to guide you. We recommend you look for a naturopath or an M.D. who is knowledgeable about nutritional or orthomolecular medicine and who is open to the use of natural, complementary options. There is a growing number of physicians who are embracing the latest research on nutrition, herbal medicine, supplementation, and complementary methods and using their knowledge to help their overweight patients.

Naturopaths take a holistic view of obesity and can provide nutritional advice, exercise programs, vitamin supplement regimens, and herbal remedies. They are the only licensed primary health care practitioners who receive comprehensive training in therapeutic diets and preventive nutrition, as well as comprehensive training in behavior-oriented counseling. Naturopaths complete their four-year doctoral program at one of three naturopathic medical schools in the United States and are bestowed with a Doctor of Naturopathic Medicine (N.D.) degree.

You may elect to consult with a nutritionist. A nutritionist who is an M.D. is probably your safest choice. Not all nutritionists receive the same training: they can have one or more degrees (B.S., M.S., Ph.D.), or they may be self-styled practitioners who received their diplomas from mail-order colleges. Check the credentials of any health care provider you are considering.

Ideally, the medical professional you choose will conduct the evaluations and tests discussed later in this chapter. She or he will help you develop a healthy eating plan that addresses any allergies or medical conditions uncovered during testing as well as one that you can live with for the rest of your life. Your physician will also be involved in helping you establish an enjoyable and effective exercise program. If you choose some complementary approaches, your physician may be able to refer you to other providers, or refer to Appendix A for the names of organizations that can refer you. Some of these professionals are discussed in the next section.

Beware of family physicians, general practitioners, psychiatrists, and internists who prescribe appetite suppressants or who market special diet foods, liquid diets, or shots. Some of these individuals may list themselves as members of the American Society of Bariatric Physicians, an organization of doctors who treat obesity. "Bariatrics" has not been recognized as a legitimate specialty by the American Medical Association, and there is no certification process required to belong to this group.

Finding Natural and Complementary Medicine Providers

After you have seen your primary health provider, you may want to explore some natural techniques to help you control food cravings, reduce stress, and improve your overall sense of well-being. How do you find natural medicine practitioners? What can they do for you? In Appendix A is a listing of

professional organizations that offer referrals and information on natural medicine organizations and practitioners.

We have divided the natural medicine providers into categories and briefly explain what to expect from each type of
approach.

Herbal and Supplemental Medicine

If you are working with a naturopath, he or she can help you
with any herbal and supplemental remedies. Many M.D.s,
however, have not fully explored this area, and may be helping you with a dietary and exercise program alone. In that
case you may want to contact an herbalist or naturopath.
Herbalists consult on the use of plants and their healing
properties. Herbal medicine is not a licensed profession in
the United States, and most herbalists are self-taught or train
with knowledgeable individuals in the field. See Appendix A
for a list of organizations you can contact for referrals and
herbal information.

Stress Reduction Therapies

The field of stress reduction and relaxation therapy is growing rapidly in popularity and in the number of options
available. For weight loss, we suggest biofeedback, hypnotherapy, meditation, and visualization/guided imagery, although there are others that may be helpful as well (see
Appendix B, Sources and Suggested Readings).

Biofeedback is usually attainable through a healing or
wellness clinic or biofeedback center. Such centers are becoming more popular and typically offer a variety of ser-
vices from massage to breathing therapy, hypnosis,
meditation, and visualization. Professional hypnotherapists
also may practice in a wellness center or independently. Beware of offers from hypnotherapists who run seminar-type
sessions in which hundreds of people gather for a hypnotic

weight-loss session. You can best learn from attending one-on-one sessions or receiving training in self-hypnosis.

Professionals who practice meditation and visualization and guided imagery are often available through healing centers or stress reduction clinics associated with teaching hospitals or natural-healing training centers. Ask for individuals who have worked specifically with weight loss. Often these organizations, as well as natural health food stores and stress reduction providers in private practice, offer an introductory session at little or no cost.

"Sense" Therapies

Individuals who practice acupuncture, acupressure, or reflexology can offer complementary methods to reduce appetite, food cravings, and binge eating. Massage is another method that can be an effective way to stimulate metabolism as well as clear the lymphatic system. Acupressure and reflexology can be done easily on your own, while acupuncture requires a professional. Check the Yellow Pages under "Acupuncture" or call a local wellness clinic or center to see if an acupuncture therapist is on staff. Appendix A can help you locate an acupuncture professional in your area. Instruction in self-massage or partner massage may be available through natural healing centers or massage training clinics, or you may contact a massage therapist who is willing to teach you and a partner the proper techniques.

Assistance with aromatherapy is available either through an aromatherapist or often with naturopaths, herbalists, or homeopaths. Like herbalists, aromatherapists are usually self-taught or have trained with professionals.

Exercise Therapy

Before you start any kind of exercise program, consult with your physician. He or she can schedule you for a stress test, if indicated, and help you develop a plan suited to your needs. If you have decided to try some more unconventional exercise, such as tai chi or yoga, we recommend you take a few classes so you can learn the proper breathing techniques and movements. Group sessions are often available and may be listed in the Yellow Pages. Other places to look for a list of classes are the bulletin boards and newsletters of health food stores, nutrition centers, and wellness clinics. Your local YWCA or YMCA, health clubs, and recreation centers may offer classes as well. See Appendix A for additional sources of professionals and information on tai chi and yoga.

One thing you will find in the field of holistic health is that often there is much overlap of skills among professionals. For example, naturopaths are usually knowledgeable about herbal medicine; massage therapists are often trained in reflexology; yoga practitioners usually teach and practice breathing techniques and meditation; and hypnotherapists often use visualization during their sessions. Capitalize on these multidisciplined practitioners, because they can truly broaden your weight loss experience.

Your First Visit to a Physician

When you make the telephone call to set up your first appointment, you will likely be asked to keep a diary of your food intake for one week before your visit. The diary should include all foods and beverages consumed and their amounts, as well as time of day they were consumed. Include water, alcohol, and any medications—prescription, over-the-counter, or recreational. Be honest! The only way you will lose weight and keep it off is to give it your full commitment. Soon the new habits you will develop will become second nature. If you exercise, include those times as well.

A food and exercise diary reveals more than how many

calories you are consuming. From it, the physician can determine the ratio of carbohydrates, protein, and fats you are currently eating, which foods could cause allergic reactions, which foods can be used as a "base" when making changes to your eating plan, and where to make modifications in your exercise program.

What Tests to Expect

In addition to a complete physical examination, your health care provider will collect information on your personal and family medical history. If you are 45 years or older, an electrocardiogram is usually recommended. Then she or he may conduct the following tests to get a holistic view of your physical condition before proceeding with a weight loss and maintenance program.

• Determine your basal metabolic rate (BMR)—the rate at which your body burns calories to maintain its functions while at rest. Factors that affect BMR include sex, age, activity level, thyroid function, amount of body fat, amount of sleep, body temperature, current weight, dietary habits, and genetics.

• A complete thyroid hormone panel to rule out low thyroid function, known as hypothyroidism, which can make losing weight difficult or impossible. The test detects the levels of thyroid hormones T-3 and T-4, which control the body's metabolic rate.

• Evaluation of digestive tract function. The test, which is called a Comprehensive Digestive Stool Analysis, provides information on the entire gastrointestinal tract, including the presence of bacteria or candida infection or toxins in the bowel, amount of stomach acid in the gut, enzyme levels, and the status of intestinal permeability (whether pieces of undigested proteins are leaking into the small bowel and then leaking into the bloodstream, which can cause immune complexes and reactions and a condition known as "leaky gut"). A poorly operating digestive system will make it difficult to lose weight.

• A 24-hour urine analysis and comprehensive blood profile may be conducted in lieu of the Comprehensive Digestive Stool Analysis to determine enzyme levels.

• A blood test that includes a regular chemical screen and a complete blood count. A special computerized analysis can now be done that uncovers the functional interrelationships among all the elements in the blood. While routine blood tests provide levels of nutrients and other substances, this special test tells how and if the elements are working together properly. It can detect subtle chemical and hormone imbalances and may eliminate the need to conduct additional tests. This test also tells how prescription and over-the-counter drugs may be affecting chemical and hormone functioning.

• Food allergy and intolerance testing. Symptoms of food allergy or intolerance include hives and rash, breathing difficulties, excessive gas, diarrhea, itchy mouth, sneezing, stomach cramps, watery eyes, and severe headache. Two types of tests are done to identify food allergy: a prick-skin test and a blood or RAST (radioallergosorbent test). The prick-skin test provides fast results and can be performed in the doctor's office. The doctor places a drop of the substance being tested on your forearm or back and pricks the skin with a needle. This allows the substance to enter the skin. If you are allergic to it, a raised wheal will form within fifteen minutes.

A RAST requires that a blood sample be sent to a laboratory where tests will be done with specific foods to determine whether you have IgE antibodies to them. Results can take about one week. Both tests are reliable, but the results are best confirmed by an *elimination diet,* which can be used to both diagnose and treat food allergy and intolerance. It involves the withdrawal of foods that are suspected of causing you to have an allergic reaction and the scheduled reintroduction of these foods, one at a time, to determine which are the culprits. It can take several months to complete and should be done under a doctor's supervision. Completion of your food diary before your visit can be helpful in identifying food allergies.

• Glucose tolerance test. This test is done to detect diabetes. Because many people who are overweight also have noninsulin-dependent diabetes, your physician may administer this test if you have not had one recently. This test is done after an overnight fast. A small amount of blood is drawn and analyzed for its blood sugar level. Normal fasting blood sugar levels are 70 to 110 mg/dL. Fasting blood-sugar levels higher than 120 mg/dL may indicate diabetes, and additional testing will be done to confirm the diagnosis.

Whether or not you choose to consult with a medical doctor, naturopath, or other natural medicine practitioners, it is good to know how to reach them if and when you decide you want some assistance with your weight loss program. Sometimes just a few words of encouragement or reassurance can make a big difference in getting the pounds off and keeping them off.

GLOSSARY

Acupressure: Healing treatment that combines the Japanese method of finger pressure and the Chinese system of acupuncture points and meridians.

Acupuncture: Healing technique that involves inserting needles into specific meridian points to restore the flow of *chi,* or vital energy.

Adrenal Glands: Two organs that sit on top of the kidneys and make and release hormones such as adrenaline (epinephrine).

Amino Acids: The building blocks of proteins. There are 20 amino acids necessary for human growth and metabolism.

Amphetamines: Central nervous system stimulants.

Anorexia: Loss of appetite. This shortened term for anorexia nervosa is a condition in which individuals, usually women, have an intense fear of becoming obese and will lose up to 25 percent or more of their original body weight.

Bariatrics: A branch of medicine that deals with the prevention, control, and treatment of obesity.

Basal Metabolic Rate: The number of calories the body needs to function while at rest.

Biofeedback: A mind-body healing approach in which people can hear or see how their body responds physically so they can learn how to consciously produce more positive or beneficial physical changes.

Blood Glucose: The primary energy source for the body's cells. It also is the main sugar the body makes from food, especially carbohydrates.

Bulimia: An eating disorder characterized by bouts of overeating followed by purging.

Candidiasis: A complex medical condition in which there is an overgrowth of the yeast *Candida albicans.*

Carbohydrates: One of the three main classes of nutrients, they are a source of energy and consist mainly of sugars and starches.

Cholesterol: A fat-like substance found in blood, muscle, liver, and other human and animal tissues. Excess cholesterol in the arteries can cause heart disease.

Chromium Picolinate: One form of the essential trace element chromium, which is highly absorbable and is thus a popular form of the supplement.

Dexfenfluramine: A diet drug related to fenfluramine that increases the level of serotonin in the brain.

Diuretic: Any substance that increases the flow of urine to help eliminate extra fluid from the body.

Endocrine Glands: Glands that release hormones into the bloodstream and have an effect on metabolism.

Ephedra: An ancient Chinese herbal remedy that is widely used as a weight loss remedy and as a treatment for allergies and other respiratory conditions.

Ephedrine: A substance derived from the plant ephedra, it is used as a stimulant and a bronchodilator.

Essential Oil: The pure, concentrated essence that is extracted from plants.

Fasting Blood Glucose Test: A technique that determines how much glucose is in the blood. The normal range for blood glucose in people without diabetes is 70 to 110 mg/dL; levels higher than 140 mg/dL usually indicate diabetes.

Fats: One of the three main classes of nutrients and a source of energy in the body. Fats come in several forms: saturated fats, found in animal products and tropical oils; polyunsaturated fats, in vegetable oils; monounsaturated fats, in olives and olive oil; and hydrogenated and partially hydrogenated fats, manufactured fats found in margarines and processed foods.

Fenfluramine: A diet drug that suppresses food cravings by increasing the amount of serotonin in the brain.

Fiber: A substance present in food plants that helps the digestive process, lowers cholesterol, and helps control blood glucose levels.

Food Allergy: Any adverse reaction by the immune system to a food product or food additive.

Food Intolerance: Also known as food sensitivity, it is a delayed adverse reaction to a food or food additive. The immune system is not involved in this type of response.

Gammalinolenic Acid (GLA): An essential fatty acid found in evening primrose oil, black currant oil, and borage. The liver normally synthesizes this acid from linolenic acid.

Glucose: A simple sugar found in the blood that is the body's main source of energy.

Glucose Tolerance Test: A test that shows how well the body deals with glucose in the blood over time; used to see if a person has diabetes. A first blood sample is taken in the morning before the person has eaten; then the person drinks a liquid that has glucose in it. After one hour, a second blood sample is taken and then, one hour later, a third.

Holistic: A concept based on the perspective that everything is connected; that the entire being or entity is greater than the sum of all its parts; and that any one or more parts of a whole has an influence on the whole.

Hormone: A chemical released by special cells that "tells" other cells what to do.

Hypnotherapy: A technique that allows people to enter an altered state of consciousness in which they are very open to suggestion. It is often used therapeutically to help change behaviors, eliminate phobias, and otherwise improve the quality of people's lives.

Hypothalamus: The hunger and appetite control center of the brain.

Insulin: A hormone produced in the pancreas that helps the body use glucose for energy.

Insulin-Dependent Diabetes Mellitus: A chronic condition in which the pancreas makes little or no insulin. Also called Type I diabetes.

Leaky Gut: A condition in which undigested proteins "leak" out of the small intestine and into the bloodstream, causing various immune responses.

Leptin: A hormone that appears to let the brain know how much fat is stored in the body. It is believed it may reduce appetite and increase metabolism.

Meditation: A broad term for any one of dozens of techniques by which you focus your attention inward to help develop spiritual, physical, and mental calm and peace.

Meridian: One of twelve invisible channels that, according to Eastern concepts, are passageways for the flow of the body's vital energy.

Metabolism: The sum of the body's physical and chemical processes that allow it to function.

Naturopaths: Health care providers who have received specific training in therapeutic diets and nutrition. Typically they are concerned with nutritional, psychological, and structural aspects of health and view all as equally important.

Neurotransmitters: Chemicals in the body that transmit messages.

Noninsulin-Dependent Diabetes Mellitus (NIDDM): Also called Type II diabetes; most common form of diabetes mellitus. People with NIDDM produce some insulin, but the body cannot use it properly.

Norepinephrine: The precursor of the hormone epinephrine, which is also known as adrenaline.

Obesity: A condition in which people have 20 percent or more excess body fat for their age, sex, height, and bone structure.

Omega-6 Fatty Acids: Acids that are essential in the production of the hormone-like substances called prostaglandins, which regulate tissue function and control all the organs in the body.

Overweight: An excess amount of body weight, which includes bone, water, fat, and muscle.

Pancreas: An organ behind the lower part of the stomach that makes insulin and enzymes that help the body digest food.

Phen-Fen: A drug combination of fenfluramine and phentermine that creates calm and satiety by increasing the serotonin level in the brain. Also called fen-phen.

Phentermine: A central nervous system stimulant that suppresses the appetite center of the brain by keeping the level of norepinephrine high.

Protein: One of the three main classes of nutrients. Proteins are found in many foods, including soy products, beans, legumes, vegetables, and animal products.

Reflexology: A healing technique in which certain sites on the body, called reflex points, are associated with nerve endings and specific organ systems. When pressed, these points can suppress appetite, promote circulation, reduce pain, and stimulate overall healing.

Serotonin: A chemical in the brain that affects mood: low levels are associated with depression while higher levels are seen with improved mood.

Set Point: A weight the body tries to maintain despite attempts or other factors that work to reduce it.

Tai Chi: A Chinese movement-based meditative exercise that promotes and maintains harmony of the body and mind.

Thermogenesis: The process by which calories are transformed into heat.

Toxicity: A poisonous reaction that occurs when people ingest an amount of a substance that is greater than they can tolerate safely.

Trans Fatty Acids: Synthetically hydrogenated vegetable oils, present in margarine and some processed foods, that block cell respiration.

Visualization: A creative mental process during which you recall or form images in your mind's eye and focus your thoughts in a positive direction in order to bring about some physical, mental, emotional, or spiritual change.

Yo-Yo Dieting: Repeated cycles of weight loss followed by a regaining of the weight, often to a level that exceeds the weight level that existed before the weight loss. Also known as weight cycling.

APPENDIX A

NATURAL HEALING: GENERAL INFORMATION
American Association of Naturopathic Physicians
601 Valley Street, Suite 105
Seattle, WA 98109
(206) 298-0126

American Holistic Health Association
PO Box 17400
Anaheim, CA
(714) 779-6152

American Holistic Medical Association
6728 Old McLean Village Dr.
McLean, VA 22101
(703) 556-9728

The American Institute of Stress
124 Park Avenue
Yonkers, NY 10703
(914) 963-1200

Information about mind-body relationships and stress in health. Publishes a monthly newsletter available to the public.

Complementary Medicine Networking and Referral Service
4649 Malvern
Tucson, AZ 85711
(520) 323-6291

Office of Alternative Medicine/National Institutes of Health
9000 Rockville Pike
Bethesda, MD 20892

Weight-Control Information Network
1 Win Way
Bethesda, MD 20892-3665
(301) 570-2177; FAX: (301) 570-2186; (800) 946-8098
Website: http://niddk.nih.gov/NutritionDocs.html
WIN is a service of the NIDDK. It assembles and disseminates information to health professionals and the general public on weight control, obesity, and nutritional disorders.

ACUPRESSURE and ACUPUNCTURE
American Academy of Medical Acupuncturists
5820 Wilshire Blvd.
Suite 500
Los Angeles, CA 90036
(213) 937-5514

American Association of Acupuncture and Oriental Medicine
433 Front Street
Catasauqua, PA 18032
(610) 266-1433

American Oriental Bodywork Therapy Association
1010 Haddonsfield-Berlin Road, Suite 408
Voorhees, NJ 08043
(609) 782-1616

ALLERGY
American Academy of Allergy, Asthma and Immunology
611 East Wells Street
Milwaukee, WI 53202
(414) 272-6071

Asthma and Allergy Foundation of America
1125 15th Street, NW, Suite 502
Washington, DC 20005
(202) 466-7643

The Food Allergy Network
10400 Eaton Place, Suite 107
Fairfax, VA 22030
(800) 929-4040

AROMATHERAPY
The Smell and Taste Treatment and Research Foundation
Water Tower Place, #990 West
845 N. Michigan Avenue
Chicago, IL 60611
(312) 938-1047

BIOFEEDBACK
Biofeedback Certification Institute of America
10200 W. 44th Ave., Suite 304
Wheatridge, CO 80033
(303) 420-2902

Life Sciences Institute of Mind/Body Health
2955 SW Wanamaker Drive, Suite B
Topeka, KS 66614

HERBAL MEDICINE
American Botanical Council
PO Box 201660
Austin, TX 78720
(800) 373-7105

Herb Society of America
9019 Kirtland-Chardon Rd.
Kirtland, OH 44094
(216) 256-0514

Herb Sources
East Earth Herb Inc
PO Box 2802
Eugene, OR 97402
(800) 827-HERB

The Herb Closet
104 Main St.
Montpelier, VT 05602
(802) 223-0888

Jean's Greens
RR 1 Box 55J
Rensselaerville, NY 12147
(315) 845-6500

Mountain Rose Herbs
PO Box 2000
Redway, CA 95560
(800) 879-3337

Nature's Way
10 Mountain Springs Parkway
Springville, UT 84663
(800) 789-1577
Available in stores.

Terra Firma Botanicals
28653 Sutherlin Lane
Eugene, OR 97405
Fresh and dried herbal extracts; massage oils; $1 catalog.

HYPNOSIS
American Society of Clinical Hypnosis
2200 E. Devon Ave., Suite 291
Des Plaines, IL 60018
(708) 297-3317
Please send SASE for information.

MASSAGE
American Massage Therapy Association
820 Davis St., Suite 100
Evanston, IL 60201
(847) 864-0123

Massage Materials
Massage Magazine
PO Box 1500
Davis, CA 95617
(916) 757-6033
Bimonthly; massage, bodywork, and related healing arts.

Medical & Sports Massage Supplies
1029 Park St.
Peekskill, NY 10566
(800) 325-7423
Catalog of massage supplies and accessories.

NUTRITION
Linus Pauling Institute of Science and Medicine
(for vitamin therapy information)
(541) 737-5075

The McDougall Program
PO Box 14039
Santa Rosa, CA 95402
(707) 576-1654

North American Vegetarian Society
PO Box 72

Dolgeville, NY 13329
(518) 568-7970

Physicians Committee for Responsible Medicine
PO Box 6322
Washington, DC 20015
(202) 686-2210

Whitaker Wellness Institute
4321 Birch Street, Suite 100
Newport Beach, CA 92660
(800) 283-4584

Nutrition Publications
The Nutrition Action Health Letter
Center for Science in the Public Interest
1875 Connecticut Avenue NW, Suite 300
Washington, DC 20009-5728
(202) 332-9111
Monthly newsletter for the general public.

Vegetarian Journal
Vegetarian Resource Group
PO Box 1463
Baltimore, MD 21203
(410) 366-8343

Vegetarian Voice
North American Vegetarian Society
PO Box 72
Dolgeville, NY 13329
(518) 568-7970
Focus: health, compassionate living, and environment; recipes.

Vegetarian Times
PO Box 570
Oak Park, IL 60303

(708) 848-8100
Monthly publication; articles on health, nutrition, and cooking.

REFLEXOLOGY
International Institute of Reflexology
PO Box 12462
St. Petersburg, FL 33733-12462
(813) 343-4811

TAI CHI
Complementary Medicine Networking and Referral Service
4649 Malvern
Tucson, AZ 85711
(520) 323-6291

VISUALIZATION
The Academy for Guided Imagery
PO Box 2070
Mill Valley, CA 94942
(800) 726-2070
For guided imagery workshops and seminars.

Center for Spiritual Awareness
PO Box 7, Lake Rabun Road
Lakemont, GA 30552
(706)782-4723

The Institute of Transpersonal Psychology
744 San Antonio Rd.
Palo Alto, CA 94303
(415) 493-4430
Imagery training; mind-body consciousness and wellness workshops.

Psycho-Acoustic Technology
4536 Genoa Circle
Virginia Beach, VA 23462
(757) 456-9487

Meditation and Visualization Tapes
The Bodymind Audio Tape Program
Jeanne Achterberg, Ph.D.
New Era Media/The Arc Group
PO Box 410685-BT
San Francisco, CA
(914) 141-0685
Audiotapes for diabetes, hypertension, general relaxation, pain,
weight loss, immune system enhancement.

Image Paths, Inc.
891 Moe Drive, Suite C
Akron, OH 44310
(800) 800-8661
The audiotape series called *Health Journeys* has guided imagery
tapes for diabetes, high blood pressure, heart disease, depression,
pain, and many other conditions.

Mind/Body Health Sciences, Inc.
393 Dixon Road
Boulder, CO 80302-7177
(303) 440-8460
Relaxation cassettes and videos by Joan and Miroslav Borysenko.

QuantumQuests
Box 98
Oakview, CA 93022
(800) 772-0090

The Source Cassette Learning System
Emmet Miller, M.D.
PO Box 6930
Auburn, CA 95604
(800) 528-2737
Tapes for relaxation, pain relief. Free catalog.

YOGA
International Association of Yoga Therapists
109 Hillside Avenue
Mill Valley, CA 94941
(415) 383-4587

Yoga Materials
Himalayan Institute of Yoga, Science and Philosophy
RR 1, Box 400
Honesdale, PA 18431
(717) 253-5551
Catalog; also publishes the magazine *Yoga International*

Samata Yoga and Health Institute
4150 Tivoli Avenue
Los Angeles, CA 90066
(310) 306-8845
Manuals, videos, and audiocassettes; also offers classes.

Total Yoga (video)
White Lotus Foundation
2500 San Marcos Pass
Santa Barbara, CA 93105
(805) 964-1944

APPENDIX B: SOURCES AND SUGGESTED READINGS

Acupuncture/Acupressure

Bauer, Cathryn. *Acupressure for Everybody.* New York: Henry Holt, 1991.

Cargill, Marie. *Acupuncture: A Viable Medical Alternative.* Westport, Conn.: Praeger, 1994.

Gach, Michael Reed. *Acupressure's Potent Points: A Guide to Self-Care for Common Ailments.* New York: Bantam, 1990.

Houston, F.M. *The Healing Benefits of Acupressure.* Rev. ed. Keats, 1994.

Kaptchuk, Ted. *The Web That Has No Weaver: Understanding Chinese Medicine.* New York: Congdon & Weed, 1993.

Kenyon, Keith, M.D. *Pressure Points: Do-It-Yourself Acupuncture Without Needles.* New York: Arco Publishing, 1984.

Lundberg, Paul. *The Book of Shiatsu.* New York: Simon & Schuster, 1992.

Marcus, Paul. *Acupuncture: A Patient's Guide.* New York: Thorsons, 1985.

———. *Thorsons Introductory Guide to Acupuncture.* London: Hammersmith, 1991.

Nickel, David J. *Acupressure for Athletes.* New York: Henry Holt, 1987.

Ohashi, Wataru. *Do-It-Yourself Shiatsu*. New York: Viking, 1992.

Serizawa, Katsusuke, M.D. *Tsubo: Vital Points for Oriental Therapy*. New York: Japan Publications, 1976.

Stux, Gabriel. *Basics of Acupuncture*. Berlin, New York: Springer-Verlag, 1988.

Thompson, Gerry. *The Shiatsu Manual*. New York: Sterling Publishing, 1994.

Aromatherapy

Berwick, Ann. *Holistic Aromatherapy*. St. Paul, MN.: Llewellyn Publications, 1994.

Cunningham, Scott. *Magical Aromatherapy*. St. Paul, MN.: Llewellyn Publications, 1989.

Hirsch, Alan R., M.D. *Dr. Hirsch's Guide to Scentsational Weight Loss*. Rockport, MA: Element Books, 1997.

Jackson, Judith. *Scentual Touch: A Personal Guide to Aromatherapy*. New York: Ballantine Books.

Price, Shirley. *Aromatherapy for Common Ailments*. New York: Simon & Schuster, 1991.

Rechelbacher, Horst. *Rejuvenation: A Wellness Guide for Women and Men*. Inner Traditions International, 1987.

Tisserand, Robert. *Aromatherapy: To Heal and Tend the Body*. Wilmot, WI: Lotus Press, 1988.

———. *The Art of Aromatherapy: The Healing and Beautifying Properties of the Essential Oils of Flowers and Herbs*. Inner Traditions International, 1987.

Wildwood, Christine. *Holistic Aromatherapy*. Thorsens, 1986.

Worwood, Valerie. *The Complete Book of Essential Oils and Aromatherapy*. New York: New World Library, 1991.

Biofeedback

Green, Elmer. *Beyond Biofeedback*. New York: Delacorte, 1977.

Sedlacek, Kurt. *The Sedlacek Technique: Finding the Calm*. New York: McGraw-Hill, 1989.

Herbal Medicine

Carroll, David. *The Complete Book of Natural Medicine*. New York: Summit Books, 1980.

Castleman, Michael. *The Healing Herbs*. Emmaus, PA: Rodale Press, 1991.

Elias, Jason and Shelagh Masline. *Healing Herbal Remedies*. New York: Dell, 1995.

Hoffman, David. *The New Holistic Herbal*. Rockport, MA.: Element Books, 1992.

Inglis, Brian, and Ruth West. *The Alternative Health Guide*. New York: Knopf, 1983.

Kloss, Jethro. *Back to Eden*. Rev. ed. Loma Linda, CA: Back to Eden Books, 1994.

Lucas, Richard M. *Miracle Medicine Herbs*. Englewood Cliffs, NJ: Prentice-Hall, 1990.

Mayell, Mark. *Off-the-Shelf Natural Health: How to Use Herbs and Nutrients to Stay Well*. New York: Bantam Books, 1995.

Mills, Simon and Steven Finando. *Alternatives in Healing*. New York: NAL Books, 1989.

Mindell, Earl, RPh, PhD. *Earl Mindell's Herb Bible*. New York: Simon & Schuster, 1992.

Moore, Michael. *Medicinal Plants of the Desert and Canyon West*. Santa Fe, NM: Museum of New Mexico Press, 1989.

Murray, Michael T., N.D. *The Healing Power of Herbs*. Rocklin, CA: Prima Publishing, 1991.

Murray, Michael T., N.D. *Natural Alternatives to Over-the-Counter and Prescription Drugs*. New York: William Morrow, 1994.

Ody, Penelope. *The Complete Medicinal Herbal*. New York: Dorling Kindersley, 1993.

Shanmugasundaram ERB, et al: Use of Gymnema sylvestre leaf extract in the control of blood glucose in insulin-dependent diabetes mellitus. *J Ethnopharmacol* 30 (1990): 281–94.

Sherman, John A., N.D. *The Complete Botanical Prescriber*. Compiled by John A. Sherman, 1993.

Stein, Diane. *All Women are Healers*. Freedom, CA: The Crossing Press, 1990.

Tierra, Lesley. *The Herbs of Life: Health and Healing Using Western and Chinese Techniques*. Freedom, CA: The Crossing Press, 1992.

Tierra, Michael, N.D. *Planetary Herbology*. Twin Lakes, WI: Lotus Light Press, 1988.

———. *The Way of Herbs*. New York: Simon & Schuster, 1990.

Trattler, Ross. *Better Health Through Natural Healing*. New York: McGraw-Hill, 1985.

Tyler, Varro E., *The Honest Herbal*. 3rd ed. Binghamton, NY: Haworth Press, 1993.

Hypnotherapy

Alman, Brian M. *Self-Hypnosis: The Complete Manual*. New York: Brunner/Mazel, 1992.

Copelan, Rachael. *How to Hypnotize Yourself and Others*. New York: Lifetime Books, 1992.

Fisher, Stanley. *Discovering the Power of Self-Hypnosis*. New York: HarperCollins, 1992.

Guyonnaud, JP. *Self-Hypnosis Step by Step*. Paris, 1989; translated by Souvenir Press, London, 1996.

Haley, Jay. *Uncommon Therapy*. New York: WW Norton, 1993.

Hilgard, Ernest. *Hypnosis: In the Relief of Pain*. New York: Brunner/Mazel, 1994.

Miller, Michael, M.D. *Therapeutic Hypnosis*. New York: Human Sciences Press, 1979.

Wallace, Benjamin. *Applied Hypnosis*. Chicago: Nelson-Hall, 1979.

Yates, John. *The Complete Book of Self-Hypnosis*. Chicago: Nelson-Hall, 1984.

Massage

Anhui Medical School, China. *Chinese Massage*. Point Roberts, WA: Hartley & Marks, 1987.

DePaoli, Carlo. *The Healing Touch of Massage*. New York: Sterling Publishing, 1995.

Inkeles, Gordon. *The Art of Sensual Massage*. New York: Simon & Schuster, 1974.

Kaptchuk, Ted. *The Web That Has No Weaver. Understanding Chinese Medicine*. Congdon & Weed, 1993.

Lidell, Lucy et al. *The Book of Massage*. New York: Simon & Schuster, 1984.

Ravald, Bertild. *The Art of Swedish Massage.* New York: E.P. Dutton, 1984.

Tappan, Frances M. *Healing Massage Techniques.* Appleton & Lange, 1988.

Meditation/Visualization

Borysenko, Joan. *Minding the Body, Mending the Mind.* Toronto/New York: Bantam Books, 1988.

———. *The Power of the Mind to Heal.* Carson CA: Hay House, 1994.

Dunham, Eileen and Cindy Cooper. *Therapeutic Relaxation and Imagery Development Manual.* Cupertino, CA: Health Horizons, 1989.

Epstein, Gerald. *Healing Visualizations.* New York: Bantam, 1989.

Fanning, Patrick. *Visualization for Change.* Oakland, CA: New Harbinger, 1988.

Fezler, William. *Creative Imagery.* New York: Simon & Schuster, 1989.

LeShan, Lawrence. *Meditating to Attain a Healthy Body Weight.* Doubleday, 1994.

Liu, Da. *The Tao of Health and Longevity.* New York: Paragon, 1991.

Lusk, Julie, ed. *30 Scripts for Relaxation, Imagery and Inner Healing.* 2 vols. Duluth: Whole Person Associates, 1992.

McDonald, Kathleen. *How to Meditate.* Boston: Wisdom Publications, 1992.

Moen, Larry, ed. *Guided Imagery.* 2 vols. Naples: United States Publishing, 1992.

Naparstek, Belleruth. *Staying Well with Guided Imagery.* New York: Time/Warner, 1994.

Ornstein, Robert and David Sobel. *The Healing Mind.* New York: Simon & Schuster, 1987.

Pelletier, Kenneth R. *Mind as Healer, Mind as Slayer.* Rev. ed. New York: Delacorte, 1992.

Rossman, Martin L., M.D. *Healing Yourself: A Step-by-Step Program for Better Health Through Imagery.* New York: Walker & Co., 1987.

Samuels, Michael, M.D. *Healing with the Mind's Eye: A Guide for*

Using Imagery and Visions for Personal Growth and Healing. New York: Simon & Schuster, 1990.

Siegel, Bernie S., M.D. *Peace, Love & Healing. Bodymind Communication and the Path to Self-Healing.* New York: Harper & Row, 1989, HarperCollins 1990.

Natural Health and Healing

Berthold-Bond, Annie. *The Green Kitchen Handbook.* New York: HarperCollins, 1997.

The Burton Goldberg Group. *Alternative Medicine: The Definitive Guide.* Puyallup, WA: Futura Medicine Publishing, 1994.

Chopra, Deepak, M.D. *Perfect Health: The Complete Mind/Body Guide.* New York: Harmony Books, 1991.

———. *Quantum Healing: Exploring the Frontiers of Body, Mind, Medicine.* Bantam Books, 1993.

Cousins, Norman. *Anatomy of an Illness as Perceived by the Patient.* New York: Norton, 1979.

———. *Head First: The Biology of Hope and the Healing Power of the Human Spirit.* New York: Viking, 1990.

Dienstfrey, Harris. *Where the Mind Meets the Body.* New York: HarperCollins, 1991.

Frahm, David and Anne. *Reclaim Your Health.* Colorado Springs, CO: Pinon Press, 1995.

Goleman, Daniel and Joel Gurin. *Mind Body Medicine: How to Use Your Mind for Better Health.* Yonkers, NY: Consumer Reports Books, 1993.

Kabat-Zinn, J. *Full Catastrophic Living: Using the Wisdom of Your Body and Mind to Face Stress, Pain, and Illness.* New York: Dell Publishing, 1990.

Marti, James. *The Alternative Health and Medicine Encyclopedia* (2nd ed.). Detroit, MI: Visible Ink Press, 1997.

Monte, Tom, et al. *World Medicine: The East West Guide to Healing Your Body.* New York: Jeremy Tarcher, 1993.

Murray, Michael T. *Natural Alternatives to Over-the-Counter and Prescription Drugs.* New York: William Morrow, 1994.

Ornstein, Robert and David Sobel. *The Healing Brain.* New York: Simon & Schuster, 1988.

————. *Healthy Pleasures.* Reading, MA: Addison-Wesley, 1990.

Pelletier, Kenneth R. *Mind as Healer, Mind as Slayer.* Rev. ed. New York: Delacorte, 1992.

Reuben, Carolyn. *Antioxidants: Your Complete Guide.* Rocklin, CA: Prima Publishing, 1995.

Siegel, Bernie, M.D. *Love, Medicine and Miracles: Lessons Learned About Self-Healing from a Surgeon's Experience with Exceptional Patients.* Boston: GK Hall, 1988.

————. *Peace, Love and Healing: Bodymind Communication and the Path to Self-Healing.* New York: Harper & Row, 1989.

Weil, Andrew, M.D. *Spontaneous Healing.* Boston: Houghton Mifflin, 1994.

Weiss, Brian, M.D. *Through Time into Healing.* New York: Simon & Schuster, 1992.

Nutrition and Recipe Books

Balch, James F., and Phyllis Balch. *Prescription for Nutritional Healing.* Garden City Park, NY: Avery Publishing Group, 1993.

Ballentine, Rudolph. *Transition to Vegetarianism: An Evolutionary Step.* Honesdale, PA: Himalayan Publishers, 1987.

Berger, Stuart M., M.D. *Dr. Berger's Immune Power Cookbook.* New York: NAL, 1986.

Colbin, Annemarie. *Food and Healing.* New York: Ballantine, 1986.

Cooper, Kenneth H., M.D. *Advanced Nutritional Therapies.* Nashville, TN: Thomas Nelson, 1996.

Diamond, Marilyn, and Donald Burton Schnell. *Fitonics for Life.* New York: Avon Books, 1996.

Gagne, Steve. *The Energetics of Food.* Santa Fe: Spiral Sciences, 1990.

Haas, Elson M., M.D. *Staying Healthy with Nutrition.* Berkeley, CA: Celestial Arts, 1992.

Klaper, Michael, M.D. *Vegan Nutrition Pure and Simple.* Maui, HI: Gentle World, 1987.

Lappe, Frances M. *Diet for a Small Planet.* Rev. ed. New York: Ballantine Books, 1975.

McDougall, John M., M.D. *McDougall's Medicine.* Piscataway, NJ: New Century, 1985.

McDougall, John A., M.D. *The McDougall Program: 12 Days to Dynamic Health.* New York: Penguin, 1991.

McDougall, John A., M.D. *The New McDougall Cookbook.* New York: NAL, 1993.

Mirkin, Gabe, M.D. *Fat Free, Flavor Full.* Boston: Little, Brown, 1995.

Ohsawa, George. *The Art of Peace.* Oroville, CA: George Ohsawa Macrobiotic Foundation, 1990.

Ornish, Dean, M.D. *Eat More, Weigh Less.* New York: HarperCollins, 1993.

Pickarski, Ron. *Friendly Foods.* Berkeley, CA: Ten Speed Press, 1991.

Pitchford, Paul. *Healing with Whole Foods: Oriental Traditions and Modern Nutrition.* Berkeley, CA: North Atlantic Books, 1993.

Robbins, John. *Diet for a New America: How Your Food Choices Affect Your Health, Happiness, and the Future of Life on Earth.* Walpole, NH: Stillpoint Publishing, 1987.

——. *May All Be Fed.* New York: Morrow, 1992; Avon, 1993.

Turner, Lisa. *Meals That Heal.* Rochester, VT: Healing Arts Press, 1996.

Wasserman, Debbie. *Simply Vegan: Quick Vegetarian Meals.* Baltimore: Vegetarian Resource Group, 1991.

Werbach, Melvyn, M.D. *Healing with Food.* New York: HarperCollins, 1993.

Reflexology

Byers, Dwight. *Better Health with Foot Reflexology.* Available through the International Institute of Reflexology, PO Box 12462, St. Petersburg, FL 33733-2462.

Carter, Mildred, and Tammy Weber. *Body Reflexology.* West Nyack, NY: Parker Publishing, 1994.

Kunz, Kevin and Barbara Kunz. *Complete Guide to Foot Reflexology.* Rev. ed. Englewood Cliffs, NJ: Prentice-Hall, 1991.

——. *Hand and Foot Reflexology: A Self-Help Guide.* Englewood Cliffs, NJ: Prentice-Hall, 1984.

Norman, Laura. *Feet First: A Guide to Foot Reflexology.* New York: Simon & Schuster, 1988.

Wills, Pauline. *The Reflexology Manual: An Easy-to-Use Illustrated Guide to the Healing Zones of the Hands and Feet.* Rochester, VT: Healing Arts Press, 1995.

Tai Chi

Clark, Barbara. *Jin Shin Acutouch: The Tai Chi of Healing Arts.* San Diego: Clark Publishing, 1987.

Knocking at the Gate of Life and Other Healing Exercises from China. Translated by Edward C. Chang. Emmaus, PA: Rodale Press, 1985.

Kuo, Simmone. *Long Life, Good Health through Tai-Chi Chuan.* Berkeley, CA: North Atlantic Books, 1991.

Parry, Robert. *Tai Chi Made Easy.* Allentown, PA: People's Medical Society, 1997.

Sutton, Nigel. *Applied Tai Chi Chuan.* London: A&C Black, 1991.

Weight Loss and Management

Aronne, Louis J., M.D. *Weigh Less, Live Longer.* New York: John Wiley, 1996.

Fraser, Laura. *Losing It: America's Obsession with Weight and the Industry That Feeds on It.* New York: Dutton, 1997.

Levine, Sheldon, M.D. *Redux Revolution.* New York: William Morrow, 1996.

McDougall, John A. *The McDougall Program for a Healthy Heart.* New York: Penguin, 1996.

Wurtman, Judith J., Ph.D. *The Serotonin Solution.* New York: Fawcett Columbine, 1996.

Yoga

Folan, Lilias. *Lilias, Yoga and Your Life.* New York: Macmillan, 1981.

Hewitt, James. *The Complete Yoga Book.* New York: Schocken Books, 1990.

Kundalini Research Institute. *Sadhana Guidelines for Kundalini Yoga Daily Practice.* Los Angeles: Arcline Publications, 1988.

Monro, Robin, et al. *Yoga for Common Ailments*. New York: Simon & Schuster, 1990.

Sivananda Yoga Vedanta Center. *Learn Yoga in a Weekend.* New York: Knopf, 1993.

INDEX

ABOUT THE AUTHOR

Deborah Mitchell is a writer and editor whose medical and health-related articles have appeared in several consumer and professional journals, including *Internal Medicine World Report, Geriatrics, Hospital Formulary, Geriatrics Medicine News & Reports,* and *Organic Digest.* She has ghostwritten or coauthored five books, including *The Good Sex Book: Recovering and Discovering Your Sexual Self* and *The Natural Health Guide to Headache Relief.* She is also the author of *Natural Medicine for Back Pain.* Deborah lives and works in Tucson, Arizona.